Recent Advances in Endovascular Neurosurgery

Editors

ELAD I. LEVY
AZAM S. AHMED
JUSTIN M. CAPPUZZO

NEUROSURGERY
CLINICS OF NORTH AMERICA

www.neurosurgery.theclinics.com

Consulting Editors
RUSSELL R. LONSER
DANIEL K. RESNICK

April 2022 • Volume 33 • Number 2

ELSEVIER

1600 John F. Kennedy Boulevard • Suite 1800 • Philadelphia, Pennsylvania, 19103-2899

http://www.theclinics.com

NEUROSURGERY CLINICS OF NORTH AMERICA Volume 33, Number 2
April 2022 ISSN 1042-3680, ISBN-13: 978-0-323-85009-4

Editor: Stacy Eastman
Developmental Editor: Ann Gielou Posedio

Neurosurgery Clinics of North America (ISSN 1042-3680) is published quarterly by Elsevier Inc., 360 Park Avenue South, New York, NY 10010-1710. Months of issue are January, April, July, and October. Business and Editorial Offices: 1600 John F. Kennedy Blvd., Suite 1800, Philadelphia, PA 19103-2899. Customer Service Office: 11830 Westline Industrial Drive, St. Louis, MO 63146. Periodicals postage paid at New York, NY, and additional mailing offices. Subscription prices are $447.00 per year (US individuals), $1,043.00 per year (US institutions), $479.00 per year (Canadian individuals), $1,074.00 per year (Canadian institutions), $556.00 per year (international individuals), $1,074.00 per year (international institutions), $100.00 per year (US students), $255.00 per year (international students), and $100.00 per year (Canadian students). International air speed delivery is included in all *Clinics* subscription prices. All prices are subject to change without notice. **POSTMASTER:** Send address changes to *Neurosurgery Clinics of North America*, Elsevier Periodicals Customer Service, 11830 Westline Industrial Drive, St. Louis, MO 63146. **Customer Service: 1-800-654-2452 (US and Canada). From outside the US and Canada, call: 1-314-453-7041. Fax: 1-314-453-5170. E-mail: JournalsCustomerService-usa@elsevier.com (for print support) and journalsonlinesupport-usa@elsevier.com (for online support).**

Reprints. For copies of 100 or more, of articles in this publication, please contact the Commercial Reprints Department, Elsevier Inc., 360 Park Avenue South, New York, NY 10010-1710. Tel. 212-633-3874; Fax: 212-633-3820; E-mail: reprints@elsevier.com.

Neurosurgery Clinics of North America is covered in *MEDLINE/PubMed (Index Medicus), EMBASE/Excerpta Medica, and Current Contents/Clinical Medicine (CC/CM).*

Contributors

CONSULTING EDITORS

RUSSELL R. LONSER, MD
Professor and Chair, Department of Neurological Surgery, The Ohio State University Wexner Medical Center, Columbus, Ohio, USA

DANIEL K. RESNICK, MD, MS
Professor and Vice Chairman, Program Director, Department of Neurosurgery, University of Wisconsin-Madison School of Medicine and Public Health, Madison, Wisconsin, USA

EDITORS

ELAD I. LEVY, MD, MBA, FACS, FAHA
Professor of Neurosurgery and Radiology, L. Nelson Hopkins MD Chairman of the Department of Neurosurgery, Jacobs School of Medicine and Biomedical Sciences, University at Buffalo' Gates Vascular Institute, Kaleida Health, Buffalo, New York, USA

AZAM S. AHMED, MD, FAANS, FACS
Departments of Neurological Surgery and Radiology, University of Wisconsin-Madison

School of Medicine and Public Health, Madison, Wisconsin, USA

JUSTIN M. CAPPUZZO, MD
Cerebrovascular Fellow, Department of Neurosurgery, Jacobs School of Medicine and Biomedical Sciences, University at Buffalo, Gates Vascular Institute, Kaleida Health Buffalo, New York, USA

AUTHORS

RAWAD ABBAS, MD
Department of Neurological Surgery, Thomas Jefferson University Hospital, Philadelphia, Pennsylvania, USA

ISAAC JOSH ABECASSIS, MD
Department of Neurological Surgery, University of Louisville, Louisville, Kentucky, USA

MOHAMED ABOUELLEIL, MD
Spectrum Health Neurosurgery Resident, PYG-2, Department of Clinical Neurosciences, College of Human Medicine, Michigan State University, Department of Neurological Surgery, Spectrum Health, Grand Rapids, Michigan, USA

FELIPE C. ALBUQUERQUE, MD
Department of Neurosurgery, Barrow Neurological Institute, St. Joseph's Hospital and Medical Center, Phoenix, Arizona, USA

PRAKASH AMBADY, MD
Department of Neurology, Oregon Health & Science University, Portland, Oregon, USA

AMMAD A. BAIG, MD
Department of Neurosurgery, Jacobs School of Medicine and Biomedical Sciences, University at Buffalo, Department of Neurosurgery, Gates Vascular Institute at Kaleida Health, University at Buffalo Neurosurgery, Buffalo, New York, USA

JACOB F. BARANOSKI, MD
Department of Neurosurgery, Barrow Neurological Institute, St. Joseph's Hospital and Medical Center, Phoenix, Arizona, USA

BERNARD R. BENDOK, MD, MSCI
Chair, Department of Neurological Surgery, William J. and Charles H. Mayo Professor, Department of Otolaryngology, Department of

Radiology, Precision Neuro-therapeutics Innovation Lab, Neurosurgery Simulation and Innovation Lab, Mayo Clinic, Phoenix, Arizona, USA

JOSHUA BURKS, MD
Department of Neurological Surgery, University of Miami, Jackson Health System, Lois Pope Life Center, Miami, Florida, USA

JOSHUA S. CATAPANO, MD
Department of Neurosurgery, Barrow Neurological Institute, St. Joseph's Hospital and Medical Center, Phoenix, Arizona, USA

BRIAN W. CHONG, MD
Department of Radiology, Mayo Clinic, Phoenix, Arizona, USA

BART M. DEMAERSCHALK, MD, MSc, FRCP(C)
Department of Neurology, Mayo Clinic, Phoenix, Arizona, USA

ANDREW F. DUCRUET, MD
Department of Neurosurgery, Barrow Neurological Institute, St. Joseph's Hospital and Medical Center, Phoenix, Arizona, USA

JEFF EHRESMAN, MD
Department of Neurosurgery, Barrow Neurological Institute, St. Joseph's Hospital and Medical Center, Phoenix, Arizona, USA

KAREEM EL NAAMANI, MD
Department of Neurological Surgery, Thomas Jefferson University Hospital, Philadelphia, Pennsylvania, USA

MICHAEL R. GOOCH, MD
Department of Neurological Surgery, Thomas Jefferson University Hospital, Philadelphia, Pennsylvania, USA

VAIDYA GOVINDARAJAN, BS
Department of Neurological Surgery, University of Miami, Jackson Health System, Lois Pope Life Center, Miami, Florida, USA

BRADLEY A. GROSS, MD
Assistant Professor, Department of Neurosurgery, University of Pittsburgh Medical Center, Pittsburgh, Pennsylvania, USA

WALDO GUERRERO, MD
Department of Neurosurgery and Brain Repair, University of South Florida, Tampa, Florida, USA

RAINYA HEATH, MS
Department of Neurological Surgery, University of Miami, Jackson Health System, Lois Pope Life Center, Miami, Florida, USA

NABEEL A. HERIAL, MD, MPH
Department of Neurological Surgery, Thomas Jefferson University Hospital, Philadelphia, Pennsylvania, USA

JOSEPH S. HUDSON, MD
Resident, Department of Neurosurgery, University of Pittsburgh Medical Center, Pittsburgh, Pennsylvania, USA

PASCAL M. JABBOUR, MD
The Angela and Richard T. Clark Distinguished Professor of Neurological Surgery, Division Chief of Neurovascular Surgery and Endovascular Neurosurgery, Department of Neurological Surgery, Thomas Jefferson University Hospital, Philadelphia, Pennsylvania, USA

ASHUTOSH P. JADHAV, MD, PhD
Department of Interventional Neurology, Barrow Neurological Institute, St. Joseph's Hospital and Medical Center, Phoenix, Arizona, USA

ARIA JAMSHIDI, MD
Department of Neurological Surgery, University of Miami, Jackson Health System, Lois Pope Life Center, Miami, Florida, USA

HUNTER KING, BA
Department of Neurological Surgery, Drexel University College of Medicine, Philadelphia, Pennsylvania, USA

CHANDAN KRISHNA, MD
Department of Neurological Surgery, Precision Neuro-therapeutics Innovation Lab, Neurosurgery Simulation and Innovation Lab, Mayo Clinic, Phoenix, Arizona, USA

MICHAEL J. LANG, MD
Assistant Professor, Department of Neurosurgery, University of Pittsburgh Medical Center, Pittsburgh, Pennsylvania, USA

ELAD I. LEVY, MD, MBA, FACS, FAHA
Professor of Neurosurgery and Radiology, L.
Nelson Hopkins MD Chairman of the
Department of Neurosurgery, Jacobs School
of Medicine and Biomedical Sciences,
University at Buffalo' Gates Vascular Institute,
Kaleida Health, Buffalo, New York, USA

EVAN LUTHER, MD
Department of Neurological Surgery, University
of Miami, Jackson Health System, Lois Pope
Life Center, Miami, Florida, USA

LEAH LYONS, PA-C
Spectrum Health Neurosurgery Physician
Assistant, Department of Clinical
Neurosciences, College of Human Medicine,
Michigan State University, Department of
Neurological Surgery, Spectrum Health, Grand
Rapids, Michigan, USA

PAUL MAZARIS, MD
Clinical Assistant Professor of Neurosurgery,
Neurosurgery Program Director (elect),
Department of Clinical Neurosciences, College
of Human Medicine, Michigan State University,
Department of Neurological Surgery, Spectrum
Health, Grand Rapids, Michigan, USA

DAVID J. MCCARTHY, MD, MS
Department of Neurological Surgery, University
of Pittsburgh Medical Center, UPMC
Presbyterian, Pittsburgh, Pennsylvania, USA

J MOCCO, MD, MS
Department of Neurosurgery, Icahn School of
Medicine at Mount Sinai Hospital, New York,
New York, USA

MAXIM MOKIN, MD, PhD
Department of Neurosurgery and Brain Repair,
University of South Florida, Tampa, Florida, USA

AHMED NADA, MD
Department of Neurological Surgery, University
of Miami, Jackson Health System, Lois Pope
Life Center, Miami, Florida, USA; Department
of Neurological Surgery, Port Said University,
Port Said, Egypt

EDWARD A. NEUWELT, MD
Departments of Neurology and Neurosurgery,
Oregon Health & Science University, Portland
Veterans Affairs Medical Center, Portland,
Oregon, USA

DEVI P. PATRA, MD, MCh, MRCSED
Department of Neurological Surgery, Precision
Neuro-therapeutics Innovation Lab,
Neurosurgery Simulation and Innovation Lab,
Mayo Clinic, Phoenix, Arizona, USA

JENNY PEIH-CHIR TSAI, MD
Department of Clinical Neurosciences, College
of Human Medicine, Michigan State University,
Department of Neurological Surgery, Spectrum
Health, Grand Rapids, Michigan, USA

ANDRES RESTREPO-OROZCO, MD
Spectrum Health Neurosurgery Resident,
PYG-3, Department of Neurological Surgery,
Spectrum Health, Department of Clinical
Neurosciences, College of Human Medicine,
Michigan State University, Grand Rapids,
Michigan, USA

ROBERT H. ROSENWASSER, MD, MBA
Department of Neurological Surgery, Thomas
Jefferson University Hospital, Philadelphia,
Pennsylvania, USA

VASU SAINI, MD
Department of Neurological Surgery, University
of Miami, Jackson Health System, Lois Pope
Life Center, Miami, Florida, USA

ADNAN H. SIDDIQUI, MD, PhD
Departments of Neurosurgery and Radiology,
Jacobs School of Medicine and Biomedical
Sciences, Department of Neurosurgery, Gates
Vascular Institute at Kaleida Health, Canon
Stroke and Vascular Research Center,
University at Buffalo, Jacobs Institute,
University at Buffalo Neurosurgery, Buffalo,
New York, USA

MICHAEL SILVA, MD
Department of Neurological Surgery, University
of Miami, Jackson Health System, Lois Pope
Life Center, Miami, Florida, USA

JUSTIN SINGER, MD
Department of Neurological Surgery, Spectrum
Health, Department of Clinical Neurosciences,
College of Human Medicine, Michigan State
University, Grand Rapids, Michigan, USA

GEORGIOS S. SIOUTAS, MD
Department of Neurological Surgery, Thomas
Jefferson University Hospital, Philadelphia,
Pennsylvania, USA

ROBERT M. STARKE, MD, MS
Department of Neurological Surgery, University of Miami, Jackson Health System, Lois Pope Life Center, Miami, Florida, USA

SHAIL THANKI, MD
Department of Neurosurgery and Brain Repair, University of South Florida, Tampa, Florida, USA

STAVROPOULA I. TJOUMAKARIS, MD
Department of Neurological Surgery, Thomas Jefferson University Hospital, Philadelphia, Pennsylvania, USA

KUTLUAY ULUC, MD
Neurosurgery, Northernlight Eastern Maine Medical Center, Bangor, Maine, USA

LEONARD VERHEY, MD, PhD
Spectrum Health Neurosurgery Resident, PGY-4, Department of Clinical Neurosciences, College of Human Medicine, Michigan State University, Department of Neurological Surgery, Spectrum Health, Grand Rapids, Michigan, USA

MUHAMMAD WAQAS, MBBS
Department of Neurosurgery, Jacobs School of Medicine and Biomedical Sciences, University at Buffalo, Department of Neurosurgery, Gates Vascular Institute at Kaleida Health, University at Buffalo Neurosurgery, Buffalo, New York, USA

KURT YAEGER, MD
Department of Neurosurgery, Icahn School of Medicine at Mount Sinai Hospital, New York, New York, USA

Contents

Preface: Recent Advances in Endovascular Neurosurgery: Pushing the Envelope   xi

Elad I. Levy, Azam S. Ahmed and Justin M. Cappuzzo

Radial Access Techniques   149

Evan Luther, Joshua Burks, David J. McCarthy, Vaidya Govindarajan, Ahmed Nada, Vasu Saini, Aria Jamshidi, Hunter King, Rainya Heath, Michael Silva, Isaac Josh Abecassis, and Robert M. Starke

> Transradial access (TRA) has gained traction in neurointerventions as studies continue to demonstrate improved access site safety and equivalent end artery effectiveness when compared with traditional transfemoral techniques. Herein, we describe the technical nuances of obtaining TRA with a focus on distal TRA, left TRA, and sheathless TRA using larger bore catheters. We also discuss various strategies to avoid access site conversion if radial artery spasm or radial anomalies are encountered and offer some solutions for forming the Simmons catheter especially when it cannot be performed in the descending aorta. Lastly, we provide some insights regarding contraindications to TRA.

Radial Access Intervention   161

Andres Restrepo-Orozco, Mohamed Abouelleil, Leonard Verhey, Leah Lyons, Jenny Peih-Chir Tsai, Paul Mazaris, and Justin Singer

> Leveraging from the interventional cardiology experience, the transradial access (TRA) for neurointervention has also started to become more used for both diagnostic and therapeutic procedures. A growing body of evidence is showing a superiority of the TRA compared with the conventional transfemoral access (TFA) in terms of access site complications (ACSs), patient satisfaction and preference, hospital length of stay, and cost. Outcomes via the transradial are noninferior, and at times superior, in select neuroendovascular procedures. Future advancements in technology with radial-specific catheters and further operator experience will aid in the full adoption of the TRA for endovascular procedures.

A Renaissance in Modern and Future Endovascular Stroke Care   169

Devi P. Patra, Bart M. Demaerschalk, Brian W. Chong, Chandan Krishna, and Bernard R. Bendok

> Acute ischemic stroke continues to be a major cause of death and disability globally. Although the concept of endovascular treatment of ischemic stroke is relatively new, current evidence from high-quality randomized trials suggests a significant improvement in the clinical outcome with mechanical thrombectomy up to 24 hours from the stroke onset. There has been a paradigm shift from medical management to mechanical thrombectomy which is now considered standard of care in eligible patients. Not surprisingly, there has been a constant effort to further improve stroke care in the last few years with a common goal of ultra-rapid intervention along with highly effective revascularization methods. Currently, it is one of the most dynamic and rapidly changing subspecialties in the field of medicine with significant advances in all aspects of acute stroke treatment starting from triage in the field to poststroke rehabilitation.

Transvenous Embolization Technique for Brain Arteriovenous Malformations   185

Muhammad Waqas, Ammad A. Baig, Elad I. Levy, and Adnan H. Siddiqui

Transvenous embolization is potentially curative for small AVMs with favorable anatomic features, such as inaccessible arterial feeders, deep location, and/or a single draining vein. Successful embolization requires the control of arterial blood flow and successful navigation of the draining vein. This allows permeation of the embolizate into the nidus. Arterial inflow may be controlled using a hypercompliant balloon or systemic hypotension. We have described the use of transvenous rapid ventricular pacing and adenosine to achieve transient controlled hypotension. This requires a multidisciplinary approach, yet provides high chances of complete obliteration of the AVM.

Treatment of Spinal Arteriovenous Malformation and Fistula   193

Jeff Ehresman, Joshua S. Catapano, Jacob F. Baranoski, Ashutosh P. Jadhav, Andrew F. Ducruet, and Felipe C. Albuquerque

With the rapid advancements in endovascular therapy over previous decades, the treatment of spinal arteriovenous malformations (AVMs) continues to evolve. The decision to use endovascular versus surgical therapy largely depends on the type of lesion and its anatomic location. Recent studies demonstrate that endovascular treatment is effective for extradural arteriovenous fistulas (AVFs), intradural ventral (perimedullary) AVMs, and intramedullary spinal AVMs. Treatment of intradural dorsal (dural) AVFs remains largely surgical because of lower recurrence rates, although recent studies demonstrate equivocal outcomes. Extradural-intradural (juvenile) AVMs and conus AVMs remain difficult-to-treat lesions.

Treatment of Pseudotumor Cerebri (Sinus Stenosis)   207

Shail Thanki, Waldo Guerrero, and Maxim Mokin

Idiopathic intracranial hypertension, pseudotumor cerebri, and benign intracranial hypertension are terms used to describe a neurologic syndrome characterized by elevated intracranial pressure, headache, vision loss, and absence of underlying mass lesion and infection. Increased cerebrospinal fluid (CSF) production has been proposed to play a role in this condition; however, in patients with CSF hypersecretion with known causes such as choroid plexus hyperplasia, patients often develop ventriculomegaly and hydrocephalus. Classically, pseudotumor cerebri is diagnosed as a triad of headache, visual changes, and papilledema. This article discusses the role of medical and surgical management and the expanding role of venous stenting.

Novel Innovation in Flow Diversion: Surface Modifications   215

Joseph S. Hudson, Michael J. Lang, and Bradley A. Gross

Flow diversion is a mainstay of modern endovascular aneurysm treatment. Several surface-modified flow diverters have been introduced with a goal to reduce rates of in-stent thrombosis and the need for dual antiplatelet therapy. Preliminary follow-up data suggest that these now commercially available devices are noninferior with respect to rates of angiographic occlusion. These data also suggest that these devices have lower rates of stent-related ischemia. In this chapter, we explore these devices in detail and discuss clinical data regarding their efficacy. We also discuss an alternative bioactive surface modification strategy that has shown in vitro and in vivo efficacy.

Advances in Intraarterial Chemotherapy Delivery Strategies and Blood-Brain Barrier Disruption   219

Kutluay Uluc, Edward A. Neuwelt, and Prakash Ambady

Chemotherapeutics play a significant role in the management of most brain tumors. First pass effect, systemic toxicity, and more importantly, the blood-brain barrier pose significant challenges to the success of chemotherapy. Over the last 80 years, different techniques of intraarterial chemotherapy delivery have been performed in many studies but failed to become standard of care. The purpose of this article is to review the history of intraarterial drug delivery and osmotic blood-brain barrier disruption, identify the challenges for clinical translation, and identify future directions for these approaches.

Endovascular Robotic Interventions   225

Kareem El Naamani, Rawad Abbas, Georgios S. Sioutas, Stavropoula I. Tjoumakaris, Michael R. Gooch, Nabeel A. Herial, Robert H. Rosenwasser, and Pascal M. Jabbour

 Video content accompanies this article at http://www.neurosurgery.theclinics.com.

After robotic systems were approved for peripheral vascular interventions, many centers adopted this technology in treating carotid diseases. Robotic systems provide several advantages by eliminating radiation exposure and decreasing the rate of musculoskeletal injuries among interventionalists. The main disadvantage this technology poses is the lack of haptic feedback. Based on the experience of our center and several others, robotic systems have proved to be efficient, feasible, and safe when treating carotid diseases. One of the main goals of robotic systems is their future potential in remotely treating stroke patients living in rural geographic areas.

Future Directions of Endovascular Neurosurgery   233

Kurt Yaeger and J Mocco

In the last few decades, endovascular neurosurgery has progressed from treating conventional cerebrovascular pathology to expanding outside the realm of vascular neurosurgery. As technologies, techniques, and devices are developed and refined, more patients with neurologic conditions can be treated with a less-invasive endovascular approach. For pathologies such as neurodegenerative diseases or hydrocephalus, the surgical treatment paradigm is starting to change with novel endovascular innovations. We anticipate more pathologies treatable by endovascular means, as more technological progress is made.

NEUROSURGERY CLINICS OF NORTH AMERICA

FORTHCOMING ISSUES

July 2022
Pain Management
Joshua M. Rosenow and Julie G. Pilitsis, *Editors*

October 2022
Update on Open Vascular Surgery
Michael T. Lawton, *Editor*

January 2023
Chiari I Malformation
David D. Limbrick and Jeffrey Leonard, *Editors*

RECENT ISSUES

January 2022
Syndromic Neurosurgery
James A. Stadler III and Mari L. Groves, *Editors*

October 2021
Update on Motion Preservation Technologies
Domagoj Coric, *Editor*

July 2021
Current State of the Art in Spinal Cord Injury
John Hurlbert, *Editor*

SERIES OF RELATED INTEREST

Neurologic Clinics
https://www.neurologic.theclinics.com/
Neuroimaging Clinics
https://www.neuroimaging.theclinics.com/

THE CLINICS ARE AVAILABLE ONLINE!
Access your subscription at:
www.theclinics.com

Preface

Recent Advances in Endovascular Neurosurgery: Pushing the Envelope

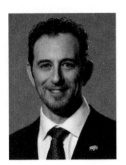

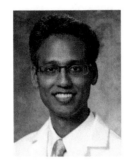

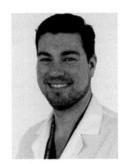

Elad I. Levy, MD, MBA, FACS, FAHA   Azam S. Ahmed, MD, FAANS, FACS,   Justin M. Cappuzzo, MD,

Editors

Neurosurgery has historically been a field that embraced rapid technological advancements. Endovascular neurosurgery is no exception to this. As we move away from traditional routes of neurosurgical therapy, we will continue to push the envelope toward less-invasive and more-innovative treatments. Many of these treatments have shortened hospital stays and have resulted in less morbidity to our patients.

We have already seen paradigm shifts in areas such as stroke, where we have been able to change the standards of care from medical management to mechanical thrombectomy, improving functional outcomes of our patients on a broad scale. For pathologic conditions not traditionally associated with endovascular treatments, such as idiopathic intracranial hypertension, we have begun to shift away from traditional techniques (cerebrospinal fluid [CSF] shunt) toward endovascular solutions, such as venous sinus stenting and novel devices that can shunt CSF from the cisterns to the venous sinuses. The latest device is a one-way valve that aims to restore normal physiology, thereby posing as a viable option for the treatment of this disease. Simultaneously, we have started exploring the role of endovascular approaches for neurooncologic therapy. Some investigators have started administering transarterial chemotherapy for diseases such as glioblastoma, with potentially promising results. Functional neurosurgery has only recently scratched the surface in terms of human-machine interfacing, with endovascular approaches now providing a minimally invasive approach to reaching cortical regions of the brain with a wireless implant in the form of a stent.

It seems that only yesterday that intracranial aneurysms were treated primarily with craniotomy for surgical clip reconstruction; however, coil embolization and flow diversion have rapidly become the standard of care for the treatment of these lesions. Now further advances, including surface modification and intrasaccular devices, have led us to administer single-antiplatelet therapy, allowing us to treat both ruptured and unruptured aneurysms with a single stent while avoiding the long-term use of dual-antiplatelet therapy. Aneurysms that were once only able to be surgically clipped can now be treated in a fraction of the time and with a much less-invasive approach.

Even access approaches within endovascular neurosurgery have seen a major change. Although femoral access was the mainstay for early endovascular access and remains a large part of our armamentarium today, alternative routes, such as transradial and transulnar access approaches, have become an important part of our everyday practice. Transvenous access, although traditionally used for central venous access for medical management, has now become an indispensable tool and the mainstay for the treatment of dural arteriovenous fistulae. Revolutionary technical advancements, such as transvenous embolization of arteriovenous malformations and rapid ventricular

Neurosurg Clin N Am 33 (2022) xi–xii
https://doi.org/10.1016/j.nec.2022.01.002
1042-3680/22/© 2022 Published by Elsevier Inc.

pacing, have augmented our therapeutic options, thereby expanding embolization from adjunct to a stand-alone curative procedure.

This is an exciting time in neurosurgery, particularly endovascular neurosurgery. It is a renaissance age within a field built on innovation. This issue of *Neurosurgery Clinics of North America* discusses some of the latest advancements in the field of endovascular neurosurgery and how technology continues to push the envelope in developing new ways for our provision of patient care.

Elad I. Levy, MD, MBA, FACS, FAHA
University at Buffalo Neurosurgery, 100 High
Street, Suite B4, Buffalo, NY 14203, USA

Azam S. Ahmed, MD, FAANS, FACS
Department of Neurological Surgery
University of Wisconsin
600 Highland Avenue
K4/850, CSC-8660
Madison, WI 53792, USA

Justin M. Cappuzzo, MD
University at Buffalo Neurosurgery, 100 High
Street, Suite B-4, Buffalo, NY 14203, USA

E-mail addresses:
elevy@ubns.com (E.I. Levy)
azam.ahmed@neurosurgery.wisc.edu
(A.S. Ahmed)
jcappuzzo@ubns.com (J.M. Cappuzzo)

Radial Access Techniques

Evan Luther, MD[a],*, Joshua Burks, MD[a], David J. McCarthy, MD, MS[b], Vaidya Govindarajan, BS[a], Ahmed Nada, MD[a,c], Vasu Saini, MD[a], Aria Jamshidi, MD[a], Hunter King, BA[d], Rainya Heath, MS[a], Michael Silva, MD[a], Isaac Josh Abecassis, MD[e], Robert M. Starke, MD, MS[a]

KEYWORDS

• Neuroendovascular • Transradial access • Long radial sheaths • Distal transradial access
• Anatomic snuffbox • Radial artery anomalies • Radial artery spasm • Access site complications

KEY POINTS

- The radial artery has become increasingly used as the primary access site in neurointerventions as results continue to demonstrate less access site complications when compared with traditional transfemoral approaches.
- Distal transradial access via the anatomic snuffbox can be more ergonomic and often allows for future procedures to be performed using standard transradial access.
- Although radial artery spasm remains one of the most frequently cited causes of access site conversion, the use of intraarterial antispasmodics among other various techniques often mitigate this risk.
- Radial artery anomalies are rare but can be navigated effectively without access site conversion if they are identified early and managed appropriately.
- Forming the Simmons catheter within the descending aorta is preferred, however, other techniques may be used when access to this location is limited anatomically.

BACKGROUND

Transradial access (TRA) was initially pioneered by interventional cardiologists after prospective studies demonstrated improved access site safety and equivalent end artery effectiveness when compared with traditional transfemoral techniques.[1–4] As the indications for endovascular treatments in neurosurgery continue to expand, a growing body of literature has also emerged evaluating the efficacy of TRA in neurointerventions.[5–8] The results of these studies seem to parallel those found in cardiology thus confirming the utility of TRA in the neuroendovascular space and solidifying this approach as a viable alternative to transfemoral access (TFA).[9–14] However, resources discussing the technical nuances of the transradial approach remain limited.[15] As such, it is the purpose of this article to provide a detailed overview of various TRA techniques and to discuss strategies that can be implemented to avoid conversion to femoral access when radial artery spasm, anatomic anomalies, and vessel tortuosity are encountered.

[a] Department of Neurological Surgery, University of Miami, Jackson Health System, Lois Pope Life Center, 2nd Floor, 1095 Northwest 14th Terrace, Miami, FL 33136, USA; [b] Department of Neurological Surgery, University of Pittsburgh Medical Center, UPMC Presbyterian, Suite B-400, 200 Lothrop Street, Pittsburgh, PA 15213, USA; [c] Department of Neurological Surgery, Port Said University, Port Fouad City, Port Said, Governorate 42526, Egypt; [d] Department of Neurological Surgery, Drexel University College of Medicine, 2900 West Queen Lane, Philadelphia, PA 19129, USA; [e] Department of Neurological Surgery, University of Louisville, 220 Abraham Flexner Way, Louisville, KY 40202, USA
* Corresponding author.
E-mail address: evan.luther@jhsmiami.org

Neurosurg Clin N Am 33 (2022) 149–159
https://doi.org/10.1016/j.nec.2021.11.003
1042-3680/22/© 2021 Elsevier Inc. All rights reserved.

DISCUSSION
Contraindications to Radial Access

As neurointerventionalists continue to gain more experience with transradial techniques, it has become more evident that there are very few absolute contraindications to TRA. In fact, the only patients in which TRA should not be attempted are those who have known anatomic arterial anomalies of the upper extremity precluding catheterization of the aortic arch or those with ipsilateral arteriovenous fistulas created for dialysis.[15] Relative contraindications include small radial artery caliber (<2 mm in diameter), anatomic anomalies of the radial artery, and radial artery occlusion. However, in each of these scenarios, techniques have been described that can allow the operator to continue the procedure transradially and will be discussed in more detail later.[16–18]

Preoperative Evaluation

Historically, many believed that preprocedural evaluation of the collateral arterial supply of the hand was necessary to avoid hand ischemia during TRA. However, studies subsequently demonstrated that these evaluations did not accurately predict periprocedural hand ischemia.[19–22] As such, most high volume transradial centers no longer perform these tests before TRA. However, it is important to review any prior imaging or angiography to determine if the patient is a good candidate for TRA. For example, if they previously had severe radial artery spasm or an aberrant right subclavian artery that would make reaching the target vessel challenging then TFA should be considered. However, prior TRA should not preclude the patient from undergoing repeat TRA especially if it was previously performed in the anatomic snuffbox as this access site has become increasingly used to mitigate the risk of more proximal radial artery occlusion.[23–25]

Patient Preparation and Positioning

Topical anesthetic cream is placed on the wrist approximately 30 minutes before the procedure. A pulse oximeter on the ipsilateral thumb is used to ensure that the patient continues to maintain proper perfusion of the hand throughout the entire case.[25] The patient is then positioned supine on the angiography table and additional local anesthetic is administered at the intended puncture site to provide further analgesia. Adequate sedation should also be provided to help reduce pain and decrease the risk of radial artery spasm.[26]

For right radial access, an extension board is used on the right side of the patient so that the right arm can remain slightly abducted and in full extension. A second support board is also placed distal to the fingertips near the knee to provide a flat surface for the proximal catheters and padding is placed along the length of the arm and on the additional support board such that the arm remains level with the rest of the body (**Fig. 1**). These maneuvers allow for a much more ergonomic working environment for the operator.[25,27]

Standard right transradial access

With the arm in the position described above, the hand is supinated with additional padding underneath the wrist to keep it extended. Tape is then used to maintain this position and provide retraction of the thenar eminence so that the radial artery near the radial styloid is exposed (**Fig. 2**).[28,29]

Right distal transradial access

Distal TRA within the anatomic snuffbox has become increasingly used in neurointerventions as studies continue to demonstrate that it reduces rates of more proximal radial artery occlusion and thus increases the rates of successful TRA in future procedures.[23–25] For this approach, the arm is again positioned in a similar manner to that seen in standard TRA. However, rather than supinating the hand, it remains more neutral with the thumb adducted and the wrist in mild ulnar deviation.[23–25] Tape is again used to maintain the hand in this position (**Fig. 3**).

Left transradial access

The overwhelming majority of transradial neuroendovascular cases are performed via the right radial artery because it is much more difficult to navigate the aortic arch and catheterize the great vessels from the left.[30–32] However, in posterior circulation cases with hypoplastic right vertebral arteries, using left TRA may provide the most direct route to the target vessel. In these cases, the left arm is placed in adduction across the patient with the elbow bent so that the left radial artery can be accessed by the operator on the right side of the patient. The left hand is often placed through the left femoral opening in the sterile drapes for ease of access. As the hand is difficult to supinate in this position, the hand is often kept pronated with the wrist in ulnar deviation so that the left anatomic snuffbox can be used for access (**Fig. 4**).[33]

Access Techniques

After positioning the upper extremity in question, the wrist and hand are prepped and draped so

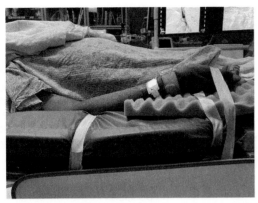

Fig. 1. Angiography table setup for right transradial access with padding underneath the arm and distal to the hand to ensure that the entire workspace is level and ergonomic.

that the puncture area remains exposed. In the awake patient, intravenous sedation is then administered. Coadministration of 50 ug of fentanyl and 1 mg of midazolam is incrementally given until the appropriate amount of sedation is achieved. As mentioned previously, local anesthetic is then injected to provide further analgesia.

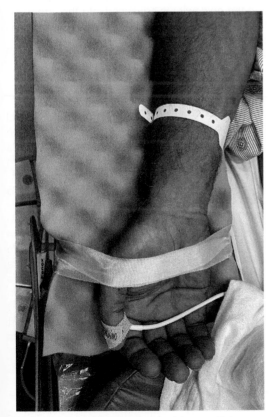

Fig. 2. Hand position for standard transradial access.

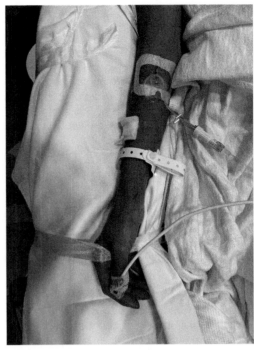

Fig. 3. Hand position for distal transradial access.

Ultrasound is then used to measure the radial artery diameter, confirm radial artery patency, and assist in arterial puncture. This is conducted in all cases as ultrasonography has been found to decrease the number of access attempts and reduce the rates of access site complications including radial artery spasm.[34]

Anatomic landmarks

In standard TRA, the radial styloid is palpated with the hand in supination (see **Fig. 2**). The radial artery is identified just proximal to the cephalad border of this bony landmark. This section of the radial artery

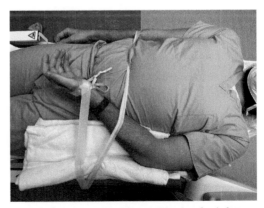

Fig. 4. Left upper extremity positioning for left transradial access.

is the preferred location for access because it is often larger in caliber and easily compressible for hemostasis. Although it can also be accessed more proximally, puncture attempts should not be performed once the artery is below the brachioradialis muscle as this impedes the ability to obtain compressive hemostasis and increases the risk of hematoma formation. This submuscular transition usually occurs 4 to 6 cm cephalad to the radial styloid.[15]

For distal TRA, the radial styloid is again palpated with the hand in a neutral position (see **Fig. 3**). The caudal border of this bony landmark identifies the proximal portion of the anatomic snuffbox. The medial and lateral borders of the snuffbox are the tendons of the extensor pollicis brevis and the extensor pollicis longus, respectively. Using these tendons as a guide, one can readily identify and access the radial artery as it passes between them.[25]

Arterial puncture and sheath placement

Once the radial artery has been identified, ultrasound is used to confirm that it is patent and then a 20-gauge needle is advanced under ultrasonography into the artery. Once the needle is intraluminal, pulsatile arterial blood should be observed exiting the needle. At this point, the operator can attempt to thread an 0.025-in guidewire through the needle into the radial artery. This is referred to as a single wall technique.[28] In TFA, a single wall puncture is typically performed as the femoral artery is of relatively large caliber and can result in unwanted hemorrhage if the needle is passed through the posterior wall of the vessel (**Fig. 5**). Given that the radial artery is a much smaller vessel, the risk of hemorrhage is

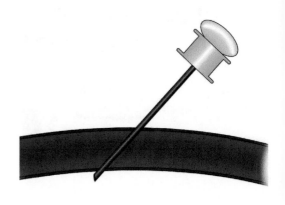

Fig. 6. Illustration demonstrating a double wall puncture technique.

significantly less, and some prefer a double-wall technique as studies have suggested it is faster and results in higher likelihood of successful radial cannulation (**Fig. 6**).[35] In the double-wall technique, the needle is advanced through the posterior wall of the radial artery after the arterial flash is encountered. The needle is then slowly withdrawn until a second arterial flash is seen at which time the guidewire is advanced into the artery. In either scenario, if an arterial flash is not encountered or if resistance is met when the guidewire is inserted into the needle, then it should not be advanced any further as it is likely extraluminal. Ultrasound should be used again to confirm the location of the needle tip and the needle should be adjusted accordingly. Alternatively, if the wire is thought to be intraluminal but resistance is felt, fluoroscopy can be performed to confirm the location of the wire. If it is truly within the radial artery it will appear straight and follow the course of the vessel within the forearm (**Fig. 7**). After the guidewire has been advanced into the radial artery, the needle can be removed and the radial sheath can be inserted over the wire into the radial artery. Special care must be taken during this step to ensure that the wire remains intraluminal but is also visible outside the proximal end of the sheath to prevent the wire from being lost in the arm (**Fig. 8**). Once the sheath is fully inserted into the arm, the guidewire and inner stylet are removed and the sheath is back bled to confirm it is intraluminal.

Radial angiography and intraprocedural medications

Once the sheath has been placed in the radial artery, intraarterial antispasmodic agents are

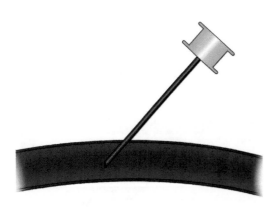

Fig. 5. Illustration demonstrating a single wall puncture technique.

administered through it to mitigate radial artery spasm. Typically 200 ug of nitroglycerin and 2.5 mg of verapamil are initially given.[15] However, these agents must be delivered slowly as they frequently cause a temporary burning sensation that is exacerbated when injected too rapidly. At this point, the AP plane should be brought in and maintained on the head side. A radial angiogram should then be performed through the sheath before advancing any catheter through it. This allows for the early identification of any radial anomalies or radial artery spasm and will help the operator confirm whether it is safe to proceed transradially. Once the decision has been made to proceed transradially, 65 to 70 units per kg of intravenous or intraarterial heparin should be administered to decrease the risk of postprocedural radial artery occlusion.[15]

Radial sheaths

Radial slender sheaths have a smaller outer diameter (OD) with the same inner diameter (ID) as their femoral counterparts which allow them to be used in a smaller caliber artery without significantly limiting the size of the catheter system. The sheaths are available in 5, 6, and 7 French (F) ODs and come in a variety of lengths ranging from 7 to 23 cm depending on the manufacturer. The 5 F sheaths are frequently used for angiograms whereas 6 or 7F are often used for interventions. However, the largest bore sheaths that can typically be used in a radial artery are 7F. For those procedures that require a larger system, a sheathless approach must be used.

Sheathless transradial access

For those cases whereby a large-bore catheter system is required, TRA should be obtained in a similar fashion to that described above. However, once the radial angiogram is obtained, a roadmap of the upper extremity should be performed. Then a 0.035-in guidewire is introduced through the sheath and navigated into the subclavian artery. Then the sheath is removed with the guidewire in place and pressure is held at the puncture site to prevent unnecessary bleeding. The guide catheter is then advanced over the wire with the inner stylet in place under fluoroscopic guidance until the stylet has reached the subclavian artery. Special attention again should be paid to the wire during this step so that it is not inadvertently advanced more proximally into the arch. As such, wire should be seen exiting the proximal end of the guide catheter before advancing the system into the arm. Once the catheter is in place, the wire and stylet are removed and the catheter is back bled. Most radial arteries can accommodate 8F OD guide

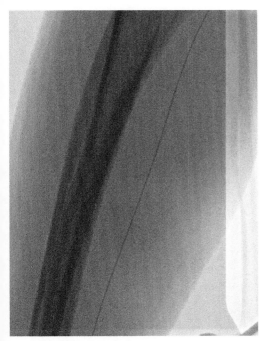

Fig. 7. Fluoroscopy demonstrating good position of the microwire within the radial artery.

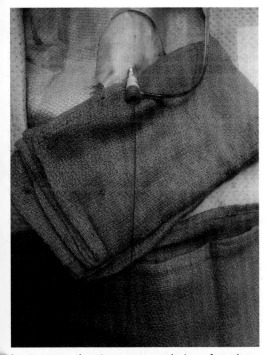

Fig. 8. Image showing proper technique for advancing the radial sheath over the microwire. Notice that there is enough wire out of the sheath to prevent it from being lost in the artery.

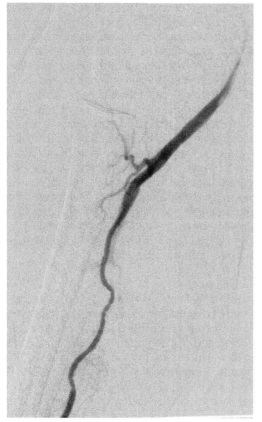

Fig. 9. Radial angiogram demonstrating significant radial artery spasm. Note the "beads-on-a-string" appearance.

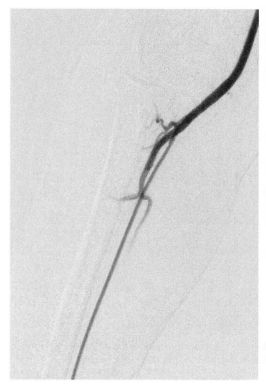

Fig. 10. Repeat radial angiogram after placement of a longer radial sheath. Note that the sheath has now bypassed the area of prior spasm.

catheters as long as the radial diameter is approximately 2 mm. If the radial artery is diminutive, alternative access sites should be considered.

Techniques to Mitigate Access Site Conversions

Despite the known benefits of TRA, radial artery spasm and radial anatomic variants remain some of the most cited reasons for transradial failures.[17,18] Furthermore, aortic arch anomalies can also present challenges to successful TRA.[36] The following sections provide an overview of strategies used to obviate the need for access site conversion when these scenarios are encountered.

Radial artery spasm

Angiographic radial artery spasm can be seen in up to 50% of patients. However, a much smaller percentage results in clinically significant stenosis that can prevent catheter movements and necessitate access site conversion (**Fig. 9**).[17] Although the manipulation of the radial artery during access

can result in vessel spasm, it can also occur due to frictional forces as the catheters are moved along the endothelium of the radial artery. As such, exchanging for a longer radial sheath when spasm is encountered often bypasses the segment of the radial artery that would be exposed to the catheter (**Fig. 10**). The 23 cm sheaths are often preferred as they typically terminate in the distal portion of the brachial artery which is of large enough caliber that the frictional forces of the catheter system are no longer at play. By implementing a protocol using these sheaths, rates of access site conversion secondary to radial artery spasm have been decreased significantly.[17]

Radial anomalies

Another frequent impetus for access site conversion is the presence of a radial anatomic variant. The 2 most common variants encountered are: (1) a radial artery loop and (2) a high brachial bifurcation. Both are congenital with the former occurring because of a tethered recurrent radial artery that forces the true radial artery into a 360° turn as the arm grows in utero (**Fig. 11**).[18] The latter is often identified by a lack of caliber change in the

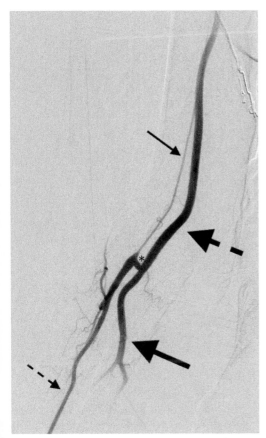

Fig. 11. Radial angiogram demonstrating a radial artery loop. Small solid arrow denotes the diminutive recurrent radial artery. Small dotted arrows denote the true radial artery. Large solid arrow denotes the ulnar artery. Large dotted arrow denotes the brachial artery. Asterisk denotes the radial loop.

radial artery whereby it typically transitions into the brachial artery at the antecubital fossa. Furthermore, the ulnar artery frequently will not opacify from a radial injection because the contrast must travel further up the arm to reach the brachial bifurcation and thus washes out before it reaches the origin of the ulnar artery (**Fig. 12**). Both of these anomalies increase the risk of developing clinically relevant radial artery spasm and in the case of a high brachial bifurcation a 23 cm sheath should be used to try to reduce the amount of exposed radial endothelium.[17] Previously, radial loops were felt to be absolute contraindications to continuing the procedure transradially. However, more recent studies have suggested that many radial loops can be navigated successfully by either circumventing the loop or catheterizing the recurrent radial artery if it is large enough or by navigating the loop with a microsystem and reducing it.[18] Only a small subset of these patients actually require access site conversion if managed appropriately.

Aortic arch abnormalities

To perform selective catheterization of the great vessels from a transradial approach, a Simmons catheter must be used. However, the Simmons catheter must be straightened when it is advanced through the upper extremity into the aortic arch. Therefore, techniques must be used to allow the catheter to regain its original shape. The most common and easiest maneuver to form the Simmons catheter is to advance it over the guidewire into the descending aorta and then gently turn the catheter while retracting the wire such that large secondary curve of the catheter falls into the ascending aorta.[36] However, tortuosity of the aortic arch frequently prevents the catheter system from being easily advanced into the descending aorta. Therefore, the selection of the common carotids or the left subclavian artery can facilitate the formation of the Simmons curve. Once these vessels are selected, the wire can be retracted and the system can be loaded forward such that the secondary curve of the catheter is formed in the arch. This is especially true in patients with bovine aortic arches whereby selection of the left common carotid occurs easily from the right subclavian artery.[36] Although there are some aortic arch anomalies that may necessitate conversion to femoral access despite implementing these strategies, even patients with an arteria lusoria can potentially undergo successful TRA. Such an anomaly results in an aberrant right subclavian artery that originates at the distal most portion of the aortic arch. Therefore, the catheter must double back on itself to select any of the great vessels. This is often identified when the Simmons catheter creates a pretzel-like appearance in the arch (**Fig. 13**). However, even in certain instances, these can be navigated successfully without issue.[37] This is typically conducted using a seesaw technique with the guidewire being advanced further into the desired great vessel than usual, followed by slow advancement of the catheter, and then further advancement of the wire until the catheter has enough purchase to maintain stability once the wire is removed.

Patent Hemostasis

At the completion of the procedure, it is imperative to maintain patent hemostasis to reduce the risk of radial artery occlusion.[38,39] Compressive, inflatable radial armbands are placed over the arteriotomy site before the removal of the final catheter

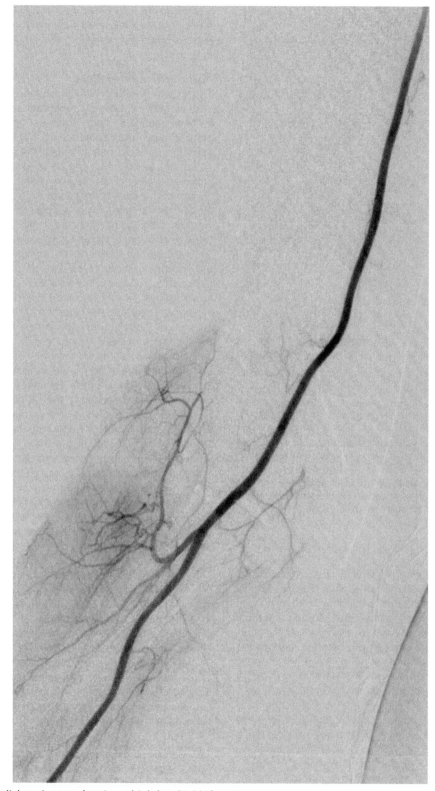

Fig. 12. Radial angiogram showing a high brachial bifurcation.

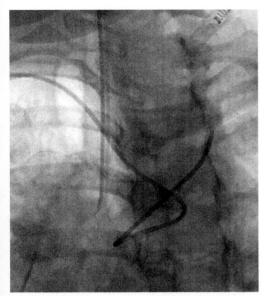

Fig. 13. Fluoroscopy demonstrating the "pretzel-like" appearance of the Simmons catheter within the aortic arch of a patient with an arteria lusoria.

or sheath. The band is then completely inflated and the system is then removed. It is then slowly deflated until bleeding is identified from the arteriotomy.[15] Then 1 to 2 cc are added to the band such that the bleeding stops. This ensures that there is enough pressure to prevent hemorrhage but that the pressure is not high enough to occlude the artery itself. The pressure in the band is then incrementally reduced over the next hour or 2 following the procedure.[15]

SUMMARY

TRA has become increasingly used in neurointerventions as results continue to demonstrate decreased access site complications when compared with transfemoral approaches with similar target vessel outcomes. Ultrasonography should be used during access to reduce failures and radial angiograms should be performed on all patients before advancing a catheter system into the radial artery. There are also very few absolute contraindications to TRA and most procedures can be completed without issue even in the presence of radial or aortic arch anomalies. Although radial artery spasm remains one of the more common causes of transradial failures, the utilization of longer radial sheaths to bypass the areas of spasm has significantly reduced rates of access site conversion in these patients.

CLINICS CARE POINTS

- TRA has less access site complications than the transfemoral approach.
- Ultrasonography during access increases rates of successful radial artery cannulation.
- Radial artery angiograms should be performed on every patient to identify radial artery spasm or any radial anomalies.
- Longer radial sheaths should be used when a patient has radial artery spasm to mitigate the risk of access site conversion.
- Radial anomalies can often be navigated and reduced successfully and are not an absolute contraindication to TRA.
- Simmons catheter formation can be performed using many different techniques and should be based on the aortic arch anatomy.
- Patent hemostasis is essential to prevent postprocedural radial artery occlusion.

ACKNOWLEDGMENTS

Roberto Suazo for creating the illustrations displayed in this article.

DISCLOSURE

The authors have nothing to disclose.

REFERENCES

1. Spaulding C, Lefevre T, Funck F, et al. Left radial approach for coronary angiography: results of a prospective study. Cathet Cardiovasc Diagn 1996; 39(4):365–70.
2. Wagener JF, Rao SV. A comparison of radial and femoral access for cardiac catheterization. Trends Cardiovasc Med 2015;25(8):707–13.
3. Aminian A, Iglesias JF, Van Mieghem C, et al. First prospective multicenter experience with the 7 French Glidesheath slender for complex transradial coronary interventions. Catheter Cardiovasc Interv 2017;89(6):1014–20.
4. Brueck M, Bandorski D, Kramer W, et al. A randomized comparison of transradial versus transfemoral approach for coronary angiography and angioplasty. JACC Cardiovasc Interv 2009; 2(11):1047–54.
5. Luther E, McCarthy DJ, Brunet MC, et al. Treatment and diagnosis of cerebral aneurysms in the post-International Subarachnoid Aneurysm Trial (ISAT)

era: trends and outcomes. J Neurointerv Surg 2020; 12(7):682–7.

6. McCarthy DJ, Diaz A, Sheinberg DL, et al. Long-term outcomes of mechanical thrombectomy for stroke: a meta-analysis. ScientificWorldJournal 2019;2019:7403104.

7. Chen CJ, Kumar JS, Chen SH, et al. Optical coherence tomography: future applications in cerebrovascular imaging. Stroke 2018;49(4):1044–50.

8. Sheinberg DL, McCarthy DJ, Elwardany O, et al. Endothelial dysfunction in cerebral aneurysms. Neurosurg Focus 2019;47(1):E3.

9. Li Y, Chen SH, Spiotta AM, et al. Lower complication rates associated with transradial versus transfemoral flow diverting stent placement. J Neurointerv Surg 2021;13(1):91–5.

10. Chen SH, Snelling BM, Sur S, et al. Transradial versus transfemoral access for anterior circulation mechanical thrombectomy: comparison of technical and clinical outcomes. J Neurointerv Surg 2019; 11(9):874–8.

11. Catapano JS, Fredrickson VL, Fujii T, et al. Complications of femoral versus radial access in neuroendovascular procedures with propensity adjustment. J Neurointerv Surg 2020;12(6):611–5.

12. Crockett MT, Selkirk GD, Chiu AH, et al. Arterial access site complications in transradial neurointerventions : single center review of 750 consecutive cases. Clin Neuroradiol 2020;30(3):639–42.

13. Maud A, Khatri R, Chaudhry MRA, et al. Transradial access results in faster skin puncture to reperfusion time than transfemoral access in posterior circulation mechanical thrombectomy. J Vasc Interv Neurol 2019;10(3):53–7.

14. Satti SR, Vance AZ, Golwala SN, et al. Patient preference for transradial access over transfemoral access for cerebrovascular procedures. J Vasc Interv Neurol 2017;9(4):1–5.

15. Jabbour PM. Radial access for neurointervention. New York, NY: Oxford University Press; 2022.

16. Babunashvili A, Dundua D. Recanalization and reuse of early occluded radial artery within 6 days after previous transradial diagnostic procedure. Catheter Cardiovasc Interv 2011;77(4):530–6.

17. Luther E, Chen S, McCarthy D, et al. Implementation of a radial long sheath protocol for radial artery spasm reduces access site conversions in neurointerventions. J Neurointerv Surg 2021;13(6):547–51.

18. Luther E, Burks J, Abecassis IJ, et al. Navigating radial artery loops in neurointerventions. J Neurointerv Surg 2021;13(11):1027–31.

19. Valgimigli M, Campo G, Penzo C, et al. Transradial coronary catheterization and intervention across the whole spectrum of Allen test results. J Am Coll Cardiol 2014;63(18):1833–41.

20. van Leeuwen MAH, Hollander MR, van der Heijden DJ, et al. The ACRA Anatomy Study (assessment of disability after coronary procedures using radial access): a comprehensive anatomic and functional assessment of the vasculature of the hand and relation to outcome after transradial catheterization. Circ Cardiovasc Interv 2017;10(11):e005753.

21. Bertrand OF, Carey PC, Gilchrist IC. Allen or no Allen: that is the question. J Am Coll Cardiol 2014; 63(18):1842–4.

22. Mason PJ, Shah B, Tamis-Holland JE, et al. An update on radial artery access and best practices for transradial coronary angiography and intervention in acute coronary syndrome: a scientific statement from the American Heart Association. Circ Cardiovasc Interv 2018;11(9):e000035.

23. Brunet MC, Chen SH, Sur S, et al. Distal transradial access in the anatomical snuffbox for diagnostic cerebral angiography. J Neurointerv Surg 2019;11(7): 710–3.

24. Chen SH, Brunet MC, Sur S, et al. Feasibility of repeat transradial access for neuroendovascular procedures. J Neurointerv Surg 2020;12(4):431–4.

25. McCarthy DJ, Chen SH, Brunet MC, et al. Distal radial artery access in the anatomical snuffbox for neurointerventions: case report. World Neurosurg 2019;122:355–9.

26. Brunet MC, Chen SH, Peterson EC. Transradial access for neurointerventions: management of access challenges and complications. J Neurointerv Surg 2020;12(1):82–6.

27. Abecassis IJ, Saini V, Phillips TJ, et al. Upper extremity transvenous access for neuroendovascular procedures: an international multicenter case series. J Neurointerv Surg 2021;13(4):357–62.

28. Layton KF, Kallmes DF, Cloft HJ. The radial artery access site for interventional neuroradiology procedures. AJNR Am J Neuroradiol 2006;27(5):1151–4.

29. Patel A, Naides AI, Patel R, et al. Transradial intervention: basics. J Vasc Interv Radiol 2015;26(5):722.

30. Al-Azizi KM, Lotfi AS. The distal left radial artery access for coronary angiography and intervention: a new era. Cardiovasc Revasc Med 2018;19(8S):35–40.

31. Barros G, Bass DI, Osbun JW, et al. Left transradial access for cerebral angiography. J Neurointerv Surg 2020;12(4):427–30.

32. Valsecchi O, Vassileva A, Cereda AF, et al. Early clinical experience with right and left distal transradial access in the anatomical snuffbox in 52 consecutive patients. J Invasive Cardiol 2018;30(6):218–23.

33. Luther E, McCarthy D, Silva M, et al. Bilateral transradial access for complex posterior circulation interventions. World Neurosurg 2020;139:101–5.

34. Seto AH, Roberts JS, Abu-Fadel MS, et al. Real-time ultrasound guidance facilitates transradial access: RAUST (Radial Artery access with Ultrasound Trial). JACC Cardiovasc Interv 2015;8(2):283–91.

35. Bernat I, Abdelaal E, Plourde G, et al. Early and late outcomes after primary percutaneous coronary

intervention by radial or femoral approach in patients presenting in acute ST-elevation myocardial infarction and cardiogenic shock. Am Heart J 2013;165(3):338–43.

36. Hadley C, Srinivasan V, Burkhardt JK, et al. Forming the simmons catheter for cerebral angiography and neurointerventions via the transradial approach-techniques and operative videos. World Neurosurg 2021;147:e351–3.

37. Jha N, Selkirk G, Crockett MT, et al. Transradial intracranial aneurysm treatment via an aberrant right subclavian artery. BMJ Case Rep 2020;13(6): e234078.

38. Pancholy SB, Bernat I, Bertrand OF, et al. Prevention of radial artery occlusion after transradial catheterization: the PROPHET-II randomized trial. JACC Cardiovasc Interv 2016;9(19):1992–9.

39. Sinha SK, Jha MJ, Mishra V, et al. Radial artery occlusion - incidence, predictors and long-term outcome after TRAnsradial Catheterization: clinico-Doppler ultrasound-based study (RAIL-TRAC study). Acta Cardiol 2017;72(3):318–27.

Radial Access Intervention

Andres Restrepo-Orozco, MD[a,b,c], Mohamed Abouelleil, MD[b,c],
Leonard Verhey, MD, PhD[b,c], Leah Lyons, PA-C[b,c], Jenny Peih-Chir Tsai, MD[b,c],
Paul Mazaris, MD[b,c], Justin Singer, MD[a,b,c],*

KEYWORDS

- Transradial access (TRA) • Transfemoral access (TFA) • Diagnostic cerebral angiogram (DCA)
- Radial first • Stroke • Mechanical thrombectomy (MT) • Aneurysm • Acute ischemic stroke

KEY POINTS

- Transradial access (TRA) for neurointervention procedures is a technically feasible, safer, and efficient alternative and with comparable outcomes to conventional transfemoral access (TFA).
- Barriers to adoption of TRA into practice are learning curve, increased fluoroscopy time, radiation exposure, and limited access-specific technology.
- There are several advantages of using the TRA over the TFA including fewer and less severe complications, increased patient satisfaction, and reduced overall health care-related costs.
- Radial-specific catheters and technology is lagging behind the technical adoption of this new approach.

INTRODUCTION

Transradial access (TRA) for neurointervention has been gaining traction in recent years due to its better safety profile and patient satisfaction as compared with conventional transfemoral access (TFA). This new paradigm shift in patient care for neurointervention procedures has been pushed forward from compelling evidence in the cardiovascular literature owing to its lower bleeding and vascular complications, patient-related outcomes, improved quality of life, and reduced cost for percutaneous coronary intervention (PCI) in acute coronary syndrome (ACS).[1] These clinical benefits have sparked our field's current interest and latest incorporation of TRA for diagnostic and neurointerventional procedures.[2–5] Despite this, neurointerventionalists have been trailing the cardiac interventionalists in the adoption of this approach, perhaps due to the lack of randomized controlled trials in our field. To this effect, operators using the TRA require a learning curve that must be overcome initially at the onset of its incorporation to practice for neuroendovascular procedures to become proficient.[5–7] Furthermore, implementation of a new approach requires a paralleled advancement in technology as robust catheter systems specifically designed for the radial approach are still lacking.[8] Nevertheless, as neuroendovascular surgeons have gained more experience in diagnostic procedures,[2,4,9] the TRA is increasingly being used for interventional procedures.[10] There is a growing body of evidence showing that the TRA has similar outcomes in neurointerventional procedures[11,12] but substantially better safety profile and patient satisfaction when compared with conventional TFA.[13] We, therefore, sought to provide an updated literature review and discussion on challenges and future directions.

BACKGROUND

Since the discovery of cerebral angiography in 1927 by Egas Moniz as the original and revolutionary imaging technique used for visualizing the

[a] Department of Neurological Surgery, Spectrum Health, Michigan State University, 25 Michigan Street Northeast, Suite 6100, Grand Rapids, MI 49503, USA; [b] Department of Clinical Neurosciences, College of Human Medicine, Michigan State University, Grand Rapids, MI, USA; [c] Department of Neurological Surgery, Spectrum Health, Grand Rapids, MI, USA
* Corresponding author. Department of Neurological Surgery, Spectrum Health, Michigan State University, 25 Michigan Street Northeast, Suite 6100, Grand Rapids, MI 49503.
E-mail address: Justin.singer@spectrumhealth.org
Twitter: @JustinSingerMD (J.S.)

Neurosurg Clin N Am 33 (2022) 161–167
https://doi.org/10.1016/j.nec.2021.11.006

cerebral vasculature and its alterations and pathologies[14]; the field of neuroendovascular surgery has come a long way. Especially remarkable is the fact that up to this point, the only means of visualizing cerebral abnormalities in a living human subject was Walter Dandy's pneumoencephalography.[15] Even more remarkable is that, for close to 50 years, cerebral angiography was the only reliable imaging modality for the investigation of intracranial disorders until the introduction of computed tomography (CT) to clinical practice.[14,16] Fast forward more than 90 years to this day today and despite the emergence multiple other imaging modalities, cerebral angiography remains indispensable, not only for the diagnosis but also for the treatment of a wealth central nervous system (CNS) disorders. From the early days of surgical and percutaneous exposure of the internal carotid artery in the early 1920s to the introduction of the Seldinger technique in 1953, the field of neuroendovascular intervention has changed significantly and has seen a dramatic increase in less invasive techniques. The TFA has traditionally dominated our field with only a scant number of case reports and case series from the early 2000s documenting their results in the literature via an alternative radial approach.[17–19] However, in the last 5 years, there has been an increment in the number of publications using the TRA for diagnostic and therapeutic neuorendovascular procedures. Perhaps a shift in paradigm was instilled to our filed from interventional cardiology due to the overwhelming evidence from numerous large prospective randomized controlled trials documenting a clear safety benefit of TRA over TFA.[1,20–23] Similarly, the Society of Neurointerventional Surgery (SNIS) has highlighted the expansion of indications for broader access options, including the role of the TRA in neurointervention.[24] Accordingly, there are now multiple large retrospective single center studies that have demonstrated its safety and efficacy.

ADVANTAGES
Lower Vascular and Overall Complications

The "radial first" strategy put forth by the AHA Scientific Statement in 2018 for PCI in ACS as an update on radial artery access and best practices marks a definitive paradigm shift in the practice of endovascular intervention.[1] Robust evidence from large international multicenter trials such as the MATRIX trial (Minimizing Adverse Haemorrhagic Events by Transradial Access Site and Systemic Implementation of AngioX) demonstrated a significantly lower rate of major bleeding (1.6% vs 2.3%; risk ratio (RR): 0.67; 95% confidence interval (CI): 0.49–0.92) and vascular complications related to surgical access site repair (0.1% vs 0.4%; $P = .0115$) in the radial access group than the femoral group. Correspondingly, the rate of major vascular complications requiring surgery was significantly lower (1.4% vs 3.7%) in the radial versus the femoral group in the RIVAL trial (radial vs femoral access for coronary intervention). Consistent with these findings are other large multicenter international trials (ACUITY, RIFLE-STEACS, STEMI_RADIAL).[20–23] However, there have been only limited retrospective studies directly comparing complication rates in the literature for neuroendovascular procedures. Some of the reported procedural-related complications are access bleeding site, hematoma formation, compartment syndrome, and arterial occlusion. Nevertheless, recent publications demonstrate a similar trend favoring a better safety profile for radial access when compared with the conventional transfemoral approach. Li and colleagues retrospectively analyzed the complication rates of TRA versus TFA for the treatment of intracranial aneurysms by flow diversion in a multicenter registry from 2010 to 2019. ACSs were more common in the femoral group (53 of 2151 cases, 2.48%) versus the radial group (0 of 134 cases, 0%) [$P = .039$]. The overall complication rate was also lower in the TRA group (3.73%) than the TFA group (9.02%, $P = .035$).[25] Similarly, Chen and colleagues found no procedural complications in 49 patients undergoing flow diversion treatment of intracranial aneurysms.[12] Conversely, Stone and colleagues found a noninferiority of the transradial approach compared with the femoral access, but found no major complications in the 2 groups and no significant statistical difference in the rate of minor complications for patients undergoing diagnostic cerebral angiograms.[26] Still, more institutions continue to report significantly higher complication rates with the TFA procedures than the TRA procedures.[27] A recent meta-analysis by Schuartz and colleagues evaluated 17 comparative studies of TRA versus TFA for neuroendovascular procedures and demonstrated that the TRA is associated with a lower incidence of ACSs but not associated with a lower rate of non-ACSs.[28] Although these results had not been explicitly examined until now, perhaps they are not all that surprising. The radial artery is a readily accessible and easily compressible vessel which makes bleeding management relatively straightforward. In addition, even in the rare instances of radial artery occlusion secondary to catheter-related manipulation, this is almost invariably a silent event and largely asymptomatic due to the rich collateral blood supply of the hand. Lower vascular and overall complication rates are not the only advantages of the radial approach.

Patient Preference and Increased Patient Satisfaction

Patient preference and increased patient satisfaction should be at the forefront of the practice of medicine. Compared with femoral artery catherization, which is more painful and uncomfortable, the alternative radial access is a more desired approach by patients undergoing neuroendovascular procedures.[4] Furthermore, patients who had experienced a prior TFA or underwent both TFA and TRA for neuroendovascular procedures had a strong preference favoring radial access as it was perceived to be less painful.[4,13] This is associated with earlier mobilization, limited bedrest, less discomfort, and shorter postprocedure recovery time which translates to improved patient satisfaction.[26]

Cost-Effectiveness

Lastly, Catapano and colleagues examined the cost of radial versus femoral access for neuroendovascular procedures in a propensity-adjusted cost analysis study.[29] They evaluated the hospital cost of 338 procedures (mainly diagnostic), (63 TRA [19%] and 275 TFA [81%]) in a single center from 2018 to 2019 and showed a significantly shorter length of hospital stay in the TRA cohort (mean (SD) 0.3 (0.5) days) compared with the TFA cohort (mean 0.7 (1.3) days; $P = .02$) and lower hospital costs (mean \$12,968 (\$6518)) compared with the TFA cohort (mean \$17,150 (\$10,946); $P = .004$) likely linked to a decreased length of hospital stay. Perhaps an even greater cost reduction would be expected if one accounts for the complication rates and their associated health-related costs.

DISADVANTAGES
Unfavorable Anatomy and Radial-Specific Complications

Although several clinical characteristics favor the TRA for neurointervention such as in obese, pregnant, and elderly patients, as well as those on oral anticoagulation; there are certain anatomic considerations that render the radial access difficult.[4] Arteria lusoria and significant subclavian or common carotid artery tortuosity significantly reduce the rate of successful cerebral catheterization and a higher crossover to TFA may be observed. In contrast, bovine aortic arch and type III aortic arch favor the TRA for most procedures. Owing to the smaller diameter of the radial artery and the lack of artery-specific catheters, another common reported barrier to the TRA adoption is the rate of radial artery spasm which can be minimized by having a preprocedural protocol that includes an antispasmodic cocktail thereby reducing the rate of crossover.[4] Accordingly, a very practical recent literature review by Brunet and colleagues identified some of the most common and uncommon challenges encountered during a TRA for DCA and neurointerventions.[30] They were able to identify challenges such as radial artery access failure, radial artery spasm, radial artery anomalies and turtosity, radial artery occlusion, radial artery perforation and hematoma, subclavian tortuosity and anomalies and catheter knots and kinks; and provided tips and tricks to help recognize and overcome those challenges thereby minimizing unnecessary morbidity and mortality.[30]

Learning Curve

Perhaps one the biggest barriers in adopting the TRA approach for neuroendovascular procedures is the operator learning curve as well as the associated inherent challenges of adjusting from traditional interventional suite set-up and team workflow. Although, many of the skills acquired for TFA are transferable to TRA, we now know form the cardiovascular literature that there is still a required minimum number of approximately 50 cases to attain a comparable outcome via the TRA with high success and low complication rates.[31,32] Tso and colleagues investigated the learning curves for TRA and TFA of 5 neuroendovascular fellows at a busy tertiary neurovascular center and found that technical proficiency improved significantly over time for both access types, normally requiring 25 to 50 DCAs to achieve asymptomatic improvement in efficiency.[33] Similarly, Zussman and colleagues reported that neurointerventionalists in a busy practice can overcome the transradial learning curve and achieve high success and low crossover rates after performing 30 to 50 cases.[6] However, in some instances, the learning curve may be longer when considering in-training personnel. Saeigh and colleagues proposed a study to compare the learning curves of TFA and TRA for diagnostic cerebral angiograms in neuroendovascular fellowship training for 2 fellows with no prior endovascular experience. A total of 293 DCA were analyzed and the fellows demonstrated a level of proficiency achieved after 60, 52, and 53 femoral cases; and 95, 77, and 64 radial cases based on fluoroscopy time, procedure time and contrast volume, respectively.[7] Despite this, safety and efficiency will continue to improve as clinicians continue to perform more of these procedures and become more familiar with catheter and access technique.[4]

Increased Fluoroscopy Times, Cross-Over Rates, Procedural Times, Radiation Exposure

Fluoroscopy time has been regarded as a metric to compare safety of vascular access in neuroendovascular procedures. Several studies have shown an increase in total fluoroscopy time via the TRA than the TFA, although this has shown not be clinically significant as radiation dose was similar between the 2 groups.[7,26] Crossover rates to the TFA and increased overall procedural times have been cited as potential barriers to the adoption of the TRA.[5,7] Certainly, it is reasonable to suggest that high volume centers with a robust operator proficiency may reduce the concerns about site crossover rates, fluoroscopy and procedural times, and overall procedural success.

Limited Technology

In addition to the lack of familiarity with the TRA, there is also hesitancy in its adoption for neuroendovascular cases due to the concern of placing larger catheters in the radial artery as well as a lack of devices with dimensions specific for radial access for interventional procedures.[10] Das and colleagues conducted a National survey within the neurointerventionalist community to look at the barriers to adoption of TRA and found that although most responders considered the TRA to technically feasible and safe, there was also a significant barrier related to catheters and equipment issues.[8] Up until now we have primarily used the technology designed and available for the femoral approach in the radial cases, which is not ideal in most cases. For instance, using a 6F system during radial artery access limits the use of larger balloon guide catheters, which have shown to be effective in stroke for mechanical thrombectomy.[5] With the current trend to transition to more radial access for neurointervention in recent years, there has been a need to create radial-specific catheters, wires and sheaths.

APPLICATIONS AND CLINICAL OUTCOMES
Diagnostic Cerebral Angiogram, Tumor Embolization, Mechanical Thrombectomy, Aneurysm Treatment, Stenting

The idea of performing DCA via a TRA has been explored since the early 2000s by Matsumoto and colleagues in a case series of 166 consecutive patients. They proposed the TRA to be considered a standard procedure as it proved to be less invasive and safer.[9] Most recently, there have been an increasing number of publications from single centers reporting their outcomes via the TRA with overall similar success rates for diagnostic purposes.[2,4–7,26,34] Similarly, the TRA for therapeutic procedures has traditionally been a reportable case.[17,18] However, in recent years the number of publications reporting their noninferior outcomes for interventional procedures has been increasing.[11,12,25,35–38] In a systematic review of 21 studies, Joshi and colleagues showed the different indications and percentages for various procedures using the TRA and demonstrated that carotid artery stenting was the most used indication (46%), followed by aneurysm treatment (32%), other nonspecified indications (11%), mechanical thrombectomy (9%), and tumor embolization (2%).[10] Similarly, a recent systematic review and meta-analysis of 7 CAS studies by Jaroenngarmsamer and colleagues, showed a high pooled procedural success outcome of 90.8% (657/723; 95% CI: 86.7%–94.2%).[37] In some instances, a 100% success rate was achieved, especially in preselected patients with favorable vascular anatomy for TRA (ie, Type III aortic arch) than the TFA.[36] A similar trend toward clinical equipoise based on clinical outcomes has been observed in acute ischemic strokes.[11,39] In a retrospective study of a cohort of 51 patients with anterior circulation strokes, Chen and colleagues demonstrated no significant differences in technical or clinical outcomes between the TRA or the TFA groups. Stroke metrics such as intraarterial recanalization after a single pass (54.5% vs 55.6%, $P = .949$), average number of passes (1.9 vs 1.7, $P = .453$), mean time from arterial access to reperfusion (61.9 vs 61.1, $P = .920$), successful revascularization (TICI $\geq$2b, 87.9% vs 88.9%, $P = 1.0$), and functional independence at discharge (modified Rankin Scale $\leq$2) was not statistically significant between the TFA and the TRA, respectively.[11] Similarly, Khanna and colleagues analyzed a single institution experience with TRA versus TFA for acute ischemic stroke in 104 (52 femoral and 52 radial) and found no significant difference in procedural and clinical outcomes in TRA compared with traditional TFA access.[39] Conversely, in a case series and meta-analysis Siddiqui and colleagues retrospectively compared TRA with TFA for acute ischemic stroke patients (222 patients, 129 TFA, and 93 TRA) and found a significantly higher rate of successful reperfusion, lower mean number of passes and higher rate of favorable functional outcomes for the TFA cohort than the TRA cohort.[40] A proposed mechanism that accounts for this difference in performance and outcomes in MT is the limited sheath size used in TRA, which restricts use of the largest aspiration catheters and balloon-guide catheters (BGC). This has traditionally been an area of criticism of TRA for stroke intervention.[40] However, a recent retrospective case series cleverly showed that the use of a sheathless 8-Fr BGC through the radial artery was safe and feasible and could potentially improve the outcomes of TRA for stroke intervention.[41] Dossani and colleagues retrospectively investigated 10 consecutive patients who had undergone MT at their institution using a highly navigable sheathless 8-Fr BGC and were able to demonstrate successful reperfusion in all cases with no ACSs, and a first pass effect (FPE) of 60%.[41] Consequently, a meta-analysis of 10 studies showed significant heterogeneity in rates of successful reperfusion[40] which could be related to procedural and technical aspects that will ultimately affect functional outcomes and mortality. These conflicting results of different institutional experiences demonstrate a need for more prospective and controlled studies before a full adoption of the TRA.

SUMMARY

The TRA for neurointervention has been increasingly used for both diagnostic and therapeutic procedures in recent years. There is a growing body of evidence is showing a clear superiority of the TRA than the conventional TFA in terms of ACSs, patient satisfaction and preference, hospital length of stay and cost. Outcomes via the transradial are noninferior, and at times superior, in select neuroendovascular procedures. Once the learning curve is overcome, the TRA shows clinical equipoise compared with the TFA. Future advancements in technology with radial-specific catheters and further operator experience will aid in the full adoption of the TRA for endovascular procedures.

CLINICS CARE POINTS

- TRA for neurointervention procedures is a technically feasible, safer, and efficient alternative and with comparable outcomes to conventional TFA

- Barriers to adoption of TRA into practice are learning curve, increased fluoroscopy time, radiation exposure, and limited access-specific technology

- There are several advantages of using the TRA over the TFA including fewer and less severe complications, increased patient satisfaction, and reduced overall health care-related costs

- Radial-specific catheters and technology is lagging behind the technical adoption of this new approach.

DISCLOSURE

The authors have nothing to disclose.

REFERENCES

1. Mason PJ, Shah B, Tamis-Holland JE, et al. An update on radial artery access and best practices for transradial coronary angiography and intervention in acute coronary syndrome: A scientific statement from the American Heart Association. Circ Cardiovasc Interv 2018;11(9):1–21.

2. Zussman BM, Tonetti DA, Stone J, et al. A prospective study of the transradial approach for diagnostic cerebral arteriography. J Neurointerv Surg 2019;1045–9. https://doi.org/10.1136/neurintsurg-2018-014686.

3. Snelling BM, Sur S, Shah SS, et al. Transradial access: Lessons learned from cardiology. J Neurointerv Surg 2018;10(5):493–8.

4. Snelling BM, Sur S, Shah SS, et al. Transradial cerebral angiography: Techniques and outcomes. J Neurointerv Surg 2018;10(9):874–81.

5. Almallouhi E, Leary J, Wessell J, et al. Fast-track incorporation of the transradial approach in endovascular neurointervention. J Neurointerv Surg 2020;12(2):176–80.

6. Zussman BM, Tonetti DA, Stone J, et al. Maturing institutional experience with the transradial approach for diagnostic cerebral arteriography: Overcoming the learning curve. J Neurointerv Surg 2019;11(12):1235–8.

7. Al Saiegh F, Sweid A, Chalouhi N, et al. Comparison of transradial vs transfemoral access in neurovascular fellowship training: overcoming the learning curve. Oper Neurosurg 2021;21(1):E3–7.

8. Das S, Ramesh S, Velagapudi L, et al. Adoption of the transradial approach for neurointerventions: a national survey of current practitioners. J Stroke Cerebrovasc Dis 2021;30(3):105589.

9. Matsumoto Y, Hongo K, Toriyama T, et al. Transradial approach for diagnostic selective cerebral angiography: Results of a consecutive series of 166 cases. AJNR Am J Neuroradiol 2001;22(4):704–8.

10. Joshi KC, Beer-Furlan A, Crowley RW, et al. Transradial approach for neurointerventions: A systematic review of the literature. J Neurointerv Surg 2020;12(9):886–92.

11. Chen SH, Snelling BM, Sur S, et al. Transradial versus transfemoral access for anterior circulation mechanical thrombectomy: Comparison of technical and clinical outcomes. J Neurointerv Surg 2019;11(9):874–8.

12. Chen SH, Snelling BM, Shah SS, et al. Transradial approach for flow diversion treatment of cerebral aneurysms: A multicenter study. J Neurointerv Surg 2019;11(8):796–800.

13. Khanna O, Sweid A, Mouchtouris N, et al. Radial artery catheterization for neuroendovascular procedures: clinical outcomes and patient satisfaction measures. Stroke 2019;50(9):2587–90.

14. Artico M, Spoletini M, Fumagalli L, et al. Egas Moniz: 90 years (1927–2017) from cerebral angiography. Front Neuroanat 2017;11:1–6.

15. Doby T. History Page Cerebral Angiography and Egas Moniz. Am J Roentgenol 1995;(August 1992): 364.

16. Riina HA. Neuroendovascular surgery. J Neurosurg 2019;131(6):1690–701.

17. Schönholz C, Nanda A, Rodriguez J, et al. Transradial approach to coil embolization of an intracranial aneurysm. J Endovasc Ther 2004;11(4):411–3.

18. Bendok BR, Przybylo JH, Parkinson R, et al. Neuroendovascular interventions for intracranial posterior circulation disease via the transradial approach: Technical case report. Neurosurgery 2005;56(3):626.

19. Levy EI, Boulos AS, Fessler RD, et al. Transradial cerebral angiography: an alternative route. Neurosurgery 2002;51(2):332–5.

20. Valgimigli M, Gagnor A, Calabró P, et al. Radial versus femoral access in patients with acute coronary syndromes undergoing invasive management: A randomised multicentre trial. Lancet 2015; 385(9986):2465–76.

21. Jolly SS, Yusuf S, Cairns J, et al. Radial versus femoral access for coronary angiography and intervention in patients with acute coronary syndromes (RIVAL): A randomised, parallel group, multicentre trial. Lancet 2011;377(9775):1409–20.

22. Romagnoli E, Biondi-Zoccai G, Sciahbasi A, et al. Radial versus femoral randomized investigation in st-segment elevation acute coronary syndrome: The rifle-steacs (radial versus femoral randomized investigation in st-elevation acute coronary syndrome) study. J Am Coll Cardiol 2012;60(24): 2481–9.

23. Bernat I, Horak D, Stasek J, et al. ST-segment elevation myocardial infarction treated by radial or femoral approach in a multicenter randomized clinical trial: The STEMI-RADIAL trial. J Am Coll Cardiol 2014;63(10):964–72.

24. Starke RM, Snelling B, Al-Mufti F, et al. Transarterial and transvenous access for neurointerventional surgery: Report of the SNIS Standards and Guidelines Committee. J Neurointerv Surg 2020;12(8): 733–41.

25. Li Y, Chen SH, Spiotta AM, et al. Lower complication rates associated with transradial versus transfemoral flow diverting stent placement. J Neurointerv Surg 2021;13(1):91–5.

26. Stone JG, Zussman BM, Tonetti DA, et al. Transradial versus transfemoral approaches for diagnostic cerebral angiography: A prospective, single-center, non-inferiority comparative effectiveness study. J Neurointerv Surg 2020;12(10):993–8.

27. Catapano JS, Fredrickson VL, Fujii T, et al. Complications of femoral versus radial access in neuroendovascular procedures with propensity adjustment. J Neurointerv Surg 2020;12(6):611–5.

28. Schartz D, Akkipeddi SMK, Ellens N, et al. Complications of transradial versus transfemoral access for neuroendovascular procedures: a meta-analysis. J Neurointerv Surg 2021. https://doi.org/10.1136/neurintsurg-2021-018032. neurintsurg-2021-018032.

29. Catapano JS, Ducruet AF, Koester SW, et al. Propensity-adjusted cost analysis of radial versus femoral access for neuroendovascular procedures. J Neurointerv Surg 2021;13(8):752–4.

30. Brunet MC, Chen SH, Peterson EC. Transradial access for neurointerventions: Management of access challenges and complications. J Neurointerv Surg 2020;12(1):82–6.

31. Hess CN, Peterson ED, Neely ML, et al. The learning curve for transradial percutaneous coronary intervention among operators in the united states: A study from the national cardiovascular data registry. Circulation 2014;129(22):2277–86.

32. Ball WT, Sharieff W, Jolly SS, et al. Characterization of operator learning curve for transradial coronary interventions. Circ Cardiovasc Interv 2011;4(4): 336–41.

33. Tso MK, Rajah GB, Dossani RH, et al. Learning curves for transradial access versus transfemoral access in diagnostic cerebral angiography: A case series. J Neurointerv Surg 2021;1–6. https://doi.org/10.1136/neurintsurg-2021-017460.

34. Brunet MC, Chen SH, Sur S, et al. Distal transradial access in the anatomical snuffbox for diagnostic cerebral angiography. J Neurointerv Surg 2019;11(7): 710–3.

35. Shapiro SZ, Sabacinski KA, Mantripragada K, et al. Access-site complications in mechanical thrombectomy for acute ischemic stroke: A review of prospective trials. AJNR Am J Neuroradiol 2020;41(3): 477–81.

36. Gao F, Lo WTJ, Sun X, et al. Selective use of transradial access for endovascular treatment of severe intracranial vertebrobasilar artery stenosis. Clin Neurol Neurosurg 2015;134:116–21.

37. Jaroenngarmsamer T, Bhatia KD, Kortman H, et al. Procedural success with radial access for carotid artery stenting: Systematic review and meta-analysis. J Neurointerv Surg 2020;12(1):87–93.

38. Khanna O, Mouchtouris N, Sweid A, et al. Transradial approach for acute stroke intervention: Technical procedure and clinical outcomes. Stroke Vasc Neurol 2020;5(1):103–6.

39. Khanna O, Velagapudi L, Das S, et al. A comparison of radial versus femoral artery access for acute stroke interventions. J Neurosurg 2021;135(3): 727–32.

40. Siddiqui AH, Waqas M, Neumaier J, et al. Radial first or patient first: A case series and meta-analysis of transradial versus transfemoral access for acute ischemic stroke intervention. J Neurointerv Surg 2021;13(8):687–92.

41. Dossani RH, Waqas M, Monteiro A, et al. Use of a sheathless 8-French balloon guide catheter (Walrus) through the radial artery for mechanical thrombectomy: technique and case series. J Neurointerv Surg 2021;(Iv). https://doi.org/10.1136/neurintsurg-2021-017868. neurintsurg-2021-017868.

A Renaissance in Modern and Future Endovascular Stroke Care

Devi P. Patra, MD, MCh, MRCSEd[a,b,c],
Bart M. Demaerschalk, MD, MSc, FRCP(C)[d], Brian W. Chong, MD[e],
Chandan Krishna, MD[a,b,c], Bernard R. Bendok, MD, MSCI[a,b,c,e,f,*]

KEYWORDS

- Mechanical thrombectomy • Stroke • Endovascular • Stentriever

KEY POINTS

- Reducing the time between the stroke symptom onset to intervention is the key to reduce irreversible brain damage.
- Telestroke with integration of AI, Mobile stroke units, Neuro ED, Direct patient transfer to angio suite are some of the important concepts that are being evaluated to optimize the stroke management workflow.
- Use of perfusion studies are helpful to assess the extent of salvageable brain tissue that might benefit from reperfusion therapy in patient presenting beyond 6 hours of symptom onset.
- Significant advancements in aspiration catheter and stent retriever designs have allowed a faster and safer reperfusion after mechanical thrombectomy.
- Telerobotics is a revolutionary concept with a possibility of mechanic thrombectomy at remote locations using endovascular robot.

INTRODUCTION

Stroke intervention with the intention to cure is a relatively new concept. Despite the fact that the history of medicine has spanned many centuries, stroke was considered to be an irreversible pathologic process until about 3 decades ago, when systemic thrombolysis showed promising evidence of clot lysis and reversal of neurologic deficits. However, no incremental progress was made until the early twenty-first century when advancement in endovascular access made mechanical thrombectomy (MT) possible. Despite that, the benefits of MT were not fully realized until 2015, when 5 landmark randomized trials consistently proved that MT significantly improves clinical outcome as compared with best medical management in patients presenting early with large vessel occlusion. These findings have resulted in a paradigm shift in acute stroke management protocols and paved the way for other clinical trials to further refine the standard of care. Although a detailed description is beyond the scope of this article, current advancements and breakthrough concepts in the endovascular management of acute ischemic stroke are summarized later in discussion.

Acute Triage and Transfer to Angiosuite

Telestroke
The use of telemedicine in stroke care (Telestroke) is a revolutionary concept that allows

Conflict of Interest: None.
[a] Department of Neurological Surgery, Mayo Clinic, 5777 East Mayo Blvd, Phoenix, AZ 85054, USA; [b] Precision Neuro-therapeutics Innovation Lab, Mayo Clinic, Phoenix, AZ, USA; [c] Neurosurgery Simulation and Innovation Lab, Mayo Clinic, Phoenix, AZ, USA; [d] Department of Neurology, Mayo Clinic, 5777 East Mayo Blvd, Phoenix, AZ 85054, USA; [e] Department of Radiology, Mayo Clinic, 5777 East Mayo Blvd, Phoenix, AZ 85054, USA; [f] Department of Otolaryngology, Mayo Clinic, Phoenix, AZ, USA
* Corresponding author. Department of Neurosurgery, 5777 E Mayo Blvd, Phoenix, AZ 85054.
E-mail address: bendok.bernard@mayo.edu

Neurosurg Clin N Am 33 (2022) 169–183
https://doi.org/10.1016/j.nec.2021.12.001
1042-3680/22/© 2021 Elsevier Inc. All rights reserved.

high-quality care by health care professionals in relatively underserved areas guided by a stroke specialist at remote hospitals through web-based audiovisual interactions.[1] The use of telestroke has increased by almost 30% of US hospitals now capable of telestroke. There is a higher likelihood of successful reperfusion therapy and lower 30-day mortality in patients with ischemic stroke who are treated in a hospital with telestroke capacity.[2] The rationale of telestroke is to rapidly identify the patients who would benefit from reperfusion therapy by timely interpreting the computed tomogram (CT) or magnetic resonance imaging (MRI) scans by a stroke expert over a teleconference. In this regard, recent advancements have been made to use artificial intelligence (AI) in image processing and interpretation through a deep machine learning algorithm. This allows rapid identification of stroke mimics (intracranial hemorrhage, mass lesions), calculation of Alberta Stroke Program Early CT score (ASPECTS), and interpretation of perfusion imaging. AI has particularly been found to be more accurate than human readers in detecting ischemic changes in patients presenting early (between 1 and 4 hours of stroke onset).[3] Integration of AI technology in telestroke has a huge potential in improving patient outcome by shortening the time delay in instituting IV thrombolysis and coordinating inter-facility transfer in patients eligible for MT.

Mobile stroke units (MSU) bring emergency hospital-grade diagnosis and treatment to the patient instead of the patient to the hospital with diagnostic capabilities such as point-of-care laboratory tests, computed tomography (CT) scanning, telemedicine capability, ride-along stroke providers, and telemedicine with the ability to rapidly deliver thrombolytic therapy.[4] MSUs have been demonstrated to be safe and effective at reducing time to thrombolysis and reducing times to therapy (decision-to treat).[5,6] With the chance to confirm the diagnosis of stroke in the field, distinguish between hemorrhagic and ischemic stroke, and screen for more severe strokes requiring a superior level of stroke care, MSUs can assist with determining whether direct transport to a comprehensive stroke center or thrombectomy capable center is best for the patient. With the high cost and limited numbers of MSUs, alternative options of including telemedicine-capable remote ambulance-based NIHSS assessment is feasible and has the potential to decrease door-to-needle times by prehospital assessment.[7] Prospective trial evidence demonstrates MSUs are capable of reducing stroke-related disability compared with standard EMS care.[8]

Direct transfer to angiosuite

The workflow in stroke care is driven by a common theme which is "Time is Brain." Timely reperfusion of the brain is an important factor associated with optimal outcome. In a retrospective study on 6756 patients, Jahan and colleagues, showed a nonlinear relationship between onset to puncture time and outcome at discharge with a steeper slope between 30 and 270 minutes as compared with more than 270 minutes.[9] In the 30 to 270 minutes time window, with every 15-min increments of faster intervention there was higher likelihood of independent ambulation at discharge. A faster endovascular treatment has also been shown to be associated with higher rate of successful reperfusion. The individual patient data meta-analysis of the HERMES group which combined the data of 7 randomized trials, showed a relative reduction of successful reperfusion (TICI 2 b/3) by 22% with every hour of delay in groin puncture since admission.[10] Therefore, a significant effort has been made to reduce the time of transfer from arrival to ED to the angiosuite with the development of dedicated stroke bay and strict institutional policies. A direct transfer to angiosuite (DTAS) method has been evaluated for eligible patients with suspected LVO within 6 hours of symptom onset to bypass the delay from initial CT/MR. Patients received a cone-beam CT in the angiosuite before angiogram to rule out hemorrhage. The median door to groin time was significantly lower in patients with DTAS as compared with standard workflow patients (16 vs 70 minutes) with a higher rate of favorable clinical outcome in the former group at 90 days (41% vs 28%).[11] More recently, a multicenter trial has been designed, WE-TRUST trial (workflow optimization to reduce time to endovascular reperfusion for ultrafast stroke treatment, NCT04701684) to further evaluate the DTAS approach.

Role of tissue plasminogen activator (tPA) in Large vessel occlusion (LVO)

The use of intravenous thrombolysis (bridging therapy) along with MT has been used as the standard therapy in patients with suspected LVO presenting within 4.5-h window. This approach has now been challenged considering the effective and rapid reperfusion achieved with MT alone. The individual patient data meta-analysis of the HERMES study showed no difference in functional independence with bridging therapy versus MT alone.[12] The SKIP trial from Japan was the initial randomized trial that evaluated the concept and failed to demonstrate the noninferiority of MT alone compared with standard bridging therapy.[13] However, 2 subsequent trials (Direct MT and DEVT trial) being conducted in China could prove the noninferiority of MT alone.[14,15] There are now 4 other trials in progress (ESTO, DIRECT SAFE, SWIFT DIRECT and MR CLEAN NO IV) evaluating the feasibility of MT alone without the use of thrombolysis (**Table 1**).

Expanding Indications for Mechanical Thrombectomy

Role of imaging

Noncontrast CT is the primary imaging modality in the evaluation of acute stroke to rule out any intracranial hemorrhage and to identify the extent of stroke seen as areas of hypodensity which are determined by the ASPECTS score. The stroke guidelines in 2015 included ASPECT score $\geq$ 6 as the imaging criteria for patients eligible for MT.[16] MRI of the brain is more sensitive and specific to detect early ischemia which seems as lesions with restricted diffusion in DWI sequences and can be seen as early as few minutes after the stroke onset. Fluid attenuated inversion recovery imaging (FLAIR) sequences also detect ischemic changes appearing as hyperintensity in the images, although it takes several hours for

this to be evident in FLAIR sequences. Therefore, DWI-FLAIR mismatch has been used as a marker to differentiate early versus late stroke to guide reperfusion therapy.[17] Because preservation of viability in brain tissue largely depends on the collateral vascular supply, patients with good collaterals can sustain brain perfusion for a longer time after a territorial occlusion. Therefore, a subset of patients may still benefit from MT even after the 6 hour time window. Perfusion imaging in this regard has been revolutionary to identify the brain parenchyma which is ischemic but without irreversible damage, hence are salvageable with timely reperfusion (penumbra). The CT or MR perfusion imaging is based on the calculation of three parameters after a bolus of contrast administration which are cerebral blood flow (CBF), cerebral blood volume (CBV), and time to peak (TTP). Overall, low CBF and CBV in an area implicate irreversible brain damage (infarct core), whereas increased TTP suggests a delay in contrast transit owing to collateral-predominant filling, leading to delay in contrast transit in that specific area. A normal CBV/CBF with increased TTP can thus identify penumbra and allow for potential

Table 1
Ongoing trials comparing direct mechanical thrombectomy to current standard of therapy (Bridging treatment with IV alteplase) in patients with large vessel occlusion

	ESTO	Direct Safe	Swift Direct	MR Clean No IV
Continent of origin	North America	Australia	Europe	Europe
Single/ multicenter	Single	Multicenter (33)	Multicenter (39)	Multicenter (20)
Number of patients	80	780	410	540
Major Inclusion criteria	• Pts $\geq$18–90 y • Within 4.5 h of onset • NIHSS $\geq$6 • Occlusion of ICA,M1,M2	• Pts $\geq$18 y • Within 4.5 h of onset • Occlusion of ICA, M1, M2, or Basilar artery	• Pts $\geq$18 y • Within 4.5 h of onset • NIHSS $\geq$5 and < 30 Occlusion of ICA, M1 • ASPECT score $\geq$4	• Pts $\geq$18 y • Within 4.5 h of onset • Occlusion of ICA, M1, M2
Major Exclusion criteria	• ASPECTS <4	• Prestroke mRS $\geq$4 • Hypodensity >1/ 3rd MCA territory	• Prestroke mRS $\geq$ 2	• Prestroke mRS $\geq$ 3
Estimated study completion date	December 2021	May 2023	December 2023	April 2022
Trial Registration Number	NCT04240470	NCT03494920	NCT03192332	ISRCTN80619088

therapeutic intervention. Most centers use CBV or CBF less than 30% of normal hemisphere as the cutoff for core infarct and a TTP threshold of more than 6 seconds as cut-off to define the penumbra. The core-penumbra mismatch is used to determine the degree of salvageable brain tissue which might benefit from reperfusion therapy. This was the basis of the recent 2 new trials (DAWN and DIFFUSE-3) on MT which evaluated the clinical benefit of MT beyond the 6-h window.[18,19] One of the notable advancements in recent years is the development of automated and semiautomated postprocessing software which provides an immediate CTA and perfusion maps and identifies the brain areas with reduced flow and vessel occlusion. One of the important benefits of these tools is the availability of mobile devices across multiple platforms, allowing rapid notification of providers within few seconds of image acquisition. These mobile applications run an automated algorithm to show the CTA map, the ASPECT score, presence or absence of large vessel occlusion, and the likelihood of candidacy for MT. There are several vender specific commercial software programs available at this time; however, the most commonly used software in the large trials including EXTEND-IA, DEFUSE 3, and DAWN trials is the rapid processing of perfusion and diffusion (RAPID) software (iSchemaView).

Leveraging the time window for mechanical thrombectomy

A revolutionary change in stroke intervention was witnessed after the success of 5 randomized trials demonstrating a significant benefit of MT in patients with large vessel occlusion.[20] In the initial guideline proposed by the American Heart Association/American Stroke Association (AHA/ASA), in 2015, the indication of MT in patients with LVO was limited to 6 hours from the stroke symptom onset.[16] With subsequent post hoc analyses from the RCTs and anecdotal reports, the benefit of MT was often observed in patients beyond the 6-h time window. With the advancement of imaging technology and use of perfusion imaging, it is now possible to identify patients with significant penumbra even after the standard 6 hours. Two important randomized trials (DIFUSE-3 and DAWN) evaluated the clinical benefit in patients after this 6-h time window.[18,19] The DEFUSE-3 trial included patients up to 16 hours, whereas the DAWN included patients up to 24 hours from symptom onset and used perfusion mismatch criteria with maximal allowable core infarct volume of 70 mL (DEFUSE-3) and 51 mL (DAWN). Both trials demonstrated improved outcome with MT in such patients beyond this 6-h time window. The

findings of these studies proved while time is an important limiting factor for stroke intervention, selected patients with preserved ischemic brain may benefit from reperfusion even if delayed. Therefore, in the new AHA/ASA guideline, the indication of MT has been expanded to include patients up to 24 hours of stroke onset provided they meet the DEFUSE-3/DAWN trial criteria.[21] There are currently 2 other trials evaluating the role of MT beyond the 6-hour time window (**Table 2**). To date, the benefit of MT beyond the 24-h window has not been evaluated in any randomized trial. In an ad hoc analysis, the DEFUSE-3 investigators found that about 20% of the patients who presented beyond 24 hours of stroke onset (so not treated with MT) continued to have mismatch for an additional 24 hours.[22] Only 10% of these patients had a favorable outcome at 90 days, suggesting that MT could have been of benefit in these patients. In another retrospective study, Desai and colleagues reviewed 21 patients who met the DAWN criteria but underwent MT beyond 24 hours of last known normal status.[23] When compared with the DAWN intervention arm, these patients had comparable clinical outcomes in terms of 90-day functional independence and safety (symptomatic intracranial hemorrhage). Currently, the evidence is insufficient to support MT in patients presenting beyond 24 hours. Randomized trials are needed to further investigate the benefits in this patient population which may allow extension of the eligibility time window for MT.

Implications of large core infarcts at presentation

Most of the RCTs evaluating the benefits of MT exclude patients with an ASPECT score less than 6 which suggests an already developed large core infarct. The HERMES group meta-analysis of 5 randomized trials shows that lower baseline ASPECTs (Less than 6) is strongly associated with lower rates of favorable outcome.[12] Similarly, in the THRACE trial, only 30% of the patients with large core infarct and poor baseline ASPECTS (0–4), had a good clinical outcome at 3 months.[24] On the other hand, a retrospective study analyzing patients with low ASPECTs (≤6) from the French Endovascular Treatment in Ischemic Stroke registry found an increased rate of favorable outcome and decreased rate of mortality in patients who had successful reperfusion with MT as compared with nonreperfused patients.[25] However, the benefit was minimal in patients with very low ASPECTS (<5) with or without reperfusion. Recently, the SELECT trial enrolling patients with large core infarcts (>50 cc on CTP) found that MT

Table 2
Ongoing trials evaluating the role of mechanical thrombectomy beyond 6 h window

	RESILIENTExt	MR Clean-Late	Tension
Continent of origin	South America	Europe	EUROPE
Single/multicenter	Multicenter	Multicenter	Multicenter
Number of patients	376	500	665
Major Inclusion Criteria	• Within 6–24 h of symptom onset • Prestroke mRS≤2 • NIHSS ≥8 • ICA or M1 occlusion	• Within 6–24 h • NIHSS ≥2 • ICA, M1/M2 occlusion	• within 12 h of stroke onset • NIHSS <26 • Prestroke mRS ≤2 • ASPECT 3–5
Major Exclusion Criteria	• ASPECT <5 • Patients receiving IV t-PA beyond 4.5 h	• Hypodensity in CT > 1/3rd of MCA territory • Patients otherwise eligible for EVT as per DAWN and DEFUSE-3 criteria	• ASPECT <3 or >5
Estimated study completion Date	May 2022	November 2022	September 2024
Trial Registration number	NCT04256096	ISRCTN19922220	NCT03094715

provides a higher rate of favorable outcome as compared with best medical management (31% vs 14%) in patients with ASPECTS score 3 to 5 with the infarct volume limited to 100 cc.[26] Several other trials have been designed to evaluate the clinical outcome in patients with large core infarcts (**Table 3**).

Role of thrombectomy in distal Middle cerebral artery (MCA) occlusions

Distal MCA region occlusions (those beyond the M1 segment) were not in the standard inclusion criteria in most of the RCTs evaluating the role of thrombectomy for large vessel occlusion. The available evidence regarding the benefit of M2 and beyond thrombectomy is based on large case series and meta-analyses. In a large retrospective case series, Sarraj and colleagues published outcomes of 288 patients undergoing thrombectomy for M2 occlusion compared with 234 patients undergoing best medical management; finding a significantly better rate of good functional outcome (90-days mRS 0–2) with thrombectomy (62.8%) versus medical management (35.4%).[27] There was a slightly higher rate of symptomatic hemorrhage with endovascular therapy (5.6% vs 2.1%); however, the difference was not significant. A meta-analysis on 12 studies with 1080 patients undergoing thrombectomy in the M2 segment showed an 81% recanalization rate comparable to M1 thrombectomies.[28] Patients with successful recanalization (TICI 2b and 3) had more than four times higher odds of

favorable outcome as compared with those with poor recanalization. Again, the risk of symptomatic intracranial hemorrhage and mortality was higher at 10% and 16%, respectively. Based on the current evidence, most of the stroke surgeons would support MT in M2 segment occlusions presenting with high NIHSS scores whereby the benefits of thrombectomy are likely to outweigh the risk of hemorrhage. Although, there have been few reports on more distal thrombectomies (M3 segments); however, considering the significant risk of hemorrhage from manipulating these small vessels with a stent it is far from the general recommendation.

Thrombectomy in tandem occlusions

Tandem lesions are defined as large vessel occlusions associated with a proximal extracranial occlusion/stenosis in the ICA or VA. Most of the randomized trials have either excluded or included only limited patients with tandem occlusions and lacked a standardized treatment strategy to address the tandem lesions. The HERMES data meta-analysis only included 122 patients with tandem lesions and found a comparable outcome in patients with tandem lesions to patients with isolated intracranial large vessel occlusions.[12] The TITAN registry investigated the effect of degree of severity of extracranial ICA lesion to procedural and clinical outcomes.[29] A lower rate of successful reperfusion (mTICI 2b-3) was noted in patients with atherosclerotic occlusions compared with those with high-grade stenosis (>90%). However,

Table 3
Ongoing trials evaluating the role of mechanical thrombectomy in patients with large ischemic core

	Select 2	Rescue-Japan Limit	Angel-Aspect	Tesla	Laste
Continent of origin	North America	Asia	Asia	North America	EUROPE
Single/multicenter	Multicenter	Multicenter	Multicenter	Multicenter	Multicenter
Number of patients	560	200	488	300	450
Major Inclusion criteria	• NIHSS ≥6 • Last known well 6–24 h • Prestroke mRS 0–1 • Large infarct core defined as ASPECT 3–5 or rCBF of <30% or ADC <620 in ≥50 cc	• NIHSS ≥6 • ASPECT 3–5 • Prestroke 0–1	• Prestroke 0–1 • NIHSS 6–30 • ASPECT 3–5 • Large infarct core defined as ASPECT 3–5 or rCBF of <30% or ADC <620 in ≥70–100 cc	• NIHSS >6 • Prestroke 0–1 • ASPECT 2–5	• Prestroke mRS 0–1 • ASPECTS 0–5 (4–5 in ≥80 yrs) • Last known normal ≤6.5 h
Major Exclusion criteria	• ASPECT ≤2 or ≥6 • tPA > 4.5 h last known normal	• Mass effect	• midline shift	• NIHSS <6 • Significant mass effect	• Significant mass effect
Estimated study completion date	November 2021	June 2021	November 2022	November 2022	February 2022
Trial Registration Number	NCT03876457	NCT03702413	NCT04551664	NCT03805308	NCT03811769

the rate of favorable outcome, procedural safety, and intracranial hemorrhage were similar. Performing thrombectomies in these situations is challenging as it involves the treatment of proximal stenosis or occlusion with stenting or angioplasty. Both an anterograde approach (which involves stenting/angioplasty of the extracranial ICA followed by distal ICA/MCA thrombectomy) and retrograde approach (initial distal access through the occluded segment and performing thrombectomy of ICA/MCA followed by the subsequent treatment of the proximal occlusion) have been reported, without any significant difference in outcome.[30] Currently, there is equivocal evidence regarding the use of carotid stenting versus angioplasty in acute settings. Proponents of carotid stenting argue that stenting allows higher recanalization rate but may entail higher risk of intracranial hemorrhage secondary to the need for postprocedural antiplatelet therapy. in a retrospective review of 95 patients, Da Ros and colleagues found a lower risk of hemorrhage with dual antiplatelet therapy in patients undergoing stenting in the index procedure; but noted an increased risk of hemorrhage with higher intraprocedural heparin dosage (≥3000 IU) when the initial ASPECTs was ≤7.[31] A multicenter randomized trial by the TITAN collaborative group is currently underway to compare the efficacy of acute ICA stenting plus MT to intracranial MT alone.[32]

Thrombectomy in posterior circulation stroke

Compared with anterior circulation stroke, the role of MT in occlusion of the vertebrobasilar system is less clearly defined. At this time, there is no definitive guideline for the treatment of posterior circulation stroke, but in general, MT is considered reasonable within 6 hours of stroke onset. Some of the unique features of posterior circulation stroke include the variability of presentation, lack of clear relation of symptom onset to the time of occlusion, and poor prognosis from brain stem stroke secondary to perforator occlusion. The BASICS registry, published before the HERMES randomized trials, evaluated the role of intra-arterial therapy (IAT) to intravenous thrombolysis (IVT) in 619 patients with posterior circulation occlusions and did not find any benefit of IAT to IVT.[33] Recently, the BASICS collaboration group randomized 300 patients with basilar occlusion to endovascular treatment with or without stenting to standard medical management with systemic thrombolysis.[34] The favorable functional outcome (mRS 0–3 at 90 days) was not statistically different between the endovascular group (44.2%) and the medical care group (37.7%). However, the study was underpowered and failed to rule out a substantial benefit of endovascular therapy over medical management.

Thrombectomy in mild stroke

The patients presenting with mild stroke score (NIHSS 0–5) are classically considered to have no large vessel occlusion or have good collateral circulation to sustain brain function, therefore, were excluded as candidates for MT. However, as high as 18% of patients with NIHSS score less than 5 and 39% of patients with NIHSS score 5 to 8 can have large vessel occlusion and therefore, may benefit from thrombectomy.[35] However, in a retrospective study of 214 patients, Sarraj and colleagues failed to demonstrate any benefit of MT in large vessel occlusions with mild strokes (NIHSS <6), while finding an increase in the rate of symptomatic intracerebral hemorrhage in patients undergoing thrombectomy as compared with medical management (5.8% vs 0%).[36] Similarly, in a recent multicenter retrospective international study which included 251 patients with mild deficit stroke (NIHSS <6), the 3-month favorable functional outcome (mRS 0–1), and functional independence (mRS 0–2) were similar between MT and best medical management. Again, the unadjusted analysis showed a higher odds of symptomatic ICH in patients undergoing thrombectomy (OR 5.52, P = .002).[37] Although, the current evidence does not support the role of MT in patients with mild stroke, a significant proportion of patients with mild stroke may develop proximal propagation of the clot and develop deterioration over time and therefore, require rescue thrombectomy. Seners and colleagues that out of 729 patients with minor stroke (NIHSS ≤5), 88 (12.1%) developed the deterioration of NIHSS score by ≥ 4 points within 24 hours. This was strongly associated with poor outcomes at 3-month irrespective of rescue thrombectomy.[38] Currently, 2 trials are underway (MOSTE and ENDO-LOW) which are evaluating the role of MT in patients with mild strokes (**Table 4**).

Thrombectomy for stroke in children, elderly and pregnant women

Although the incidence of stroke in children is low (2.3 per 100,000 children), the long-term morbidity is high. Compared with the adult population, the etiologies of stroke in children are different and major causes include congenital heart disease, sickle cell disease, and vascular disorders causing arterial dissection. Similarly, there are unique challenges in MT in the pediatric population which include small and fragile vessels, potential higher risks associated with aspiration and stent retrievers (which have not been rigorously tested in pediatric populations), as well as risks from

Table 4
Ongoing trials evaluating the role of mechanical thrombectomy in patients with mild strokes

	MOSTE	ENDOLOW
Continent of Origin	Europe	North America
Single/Multicenter	Single	Multicenter
Number of patients	824	200
Major Inclusion Criteria	• NIHSS 0–5 • ICA, M1, M2 occlusion • ASPECT ≥6 • Infarct core <70 cc • Time last known normal ≤23 h	• NIHSS 0–5 • ICA, M1 or "M1 like" M2 occlusion • ASPECT ≥6 • Infarct core <70 cc
Major Exclusion Criteria	• Prestroke mRS ≥2 • Inability to start procedure within 60 min of randomization	• Prestroke mRS ≥3 • Inability to groin puncture within 8 h of symptom onset
Estimated Study Completion date	February 2022	January 2023
Trial Registration Number	NCT03796468	NCT04167527

prolonged fluoroscopy exposure. In a multi-institutional retrospective study, Ravindra and colleagues performed 23 thrombectomies on 32 pediatric patients with a median age of 11.5 years and achieved successful recanalization (mTICI grade ≥2b) in 83% of procedures.[39] An mRS score of 0 to 2 was achieved in 86% of the patients at 90-days follow-up. Despite insufficient evidence, current recommendation from the Society of Neurointerventional Surgery (SNIS) allows MTs in eligible pediatric patients on a case by case basis.[40] Similarly, the guidelines for MT in the elderly population (age>80) is unclear and the current evidence is based on retrospective studies and post hoc analyses of randomized trials. Although the clinical benefit is worse as compared with younger patients (age<80), patients undergoing MT have an improved 90-day mRS score and 90-day mortality rate compared with those who don't. Pregnant patients pose a unique problem with a dual risk of stroke to mother and risk of intervention to mother and fetus. Specific considerations are the risk of uterine bleeding from systemic thrombolysis and risks of radiation from MT. Based on the available evidence, the SNIS recommends endovascular thrombectomy in eligible pregnant patients in a similar manner as nonpregnant patients with the use of available radiation safety features.[40]

Current Advancement of Thrombectomy Techniques

Stent design and mechanics

The concept of mechanical retrieval of the clot emerged during the early twenty-first century, although many attempts including microsnares, rheolytic thrombectomy, and lasers failed due to the lack of safety and efficacy profiles. The first device that showed promising results was the Mechanical Embolus Removal in Cerebral Ischemia (Merci) Retriever (Concentric Medical, Mountain View, CA) (**Fig. 1**A). The initial design consisted of a corkscrew-shaped nitinol wire of multiple helical loops of decreasing diameter which is unsheathed from a catheter over the clot to be captured. A single-arm trial (MERCI trial) enrolled 153 patients in which Merci retriever was used for MT and the results were compared with the control arm of another thrombolysis only trial (PROACT-II).[41] The rate of recanalization was 48% in patients undergoing Merci clot retrieval versus 18% as reported in PROACT-II controls. A higher proportion of patients who had successful recanalization had a good outcome at 90 days compared with the control group (46% vs 10%, $P < .0001$). Unfortunately, the reported mortality in the Merci trial was high (32%). Although the device was granted FDA approval, the safety of the device was of significant concern. Subsequently, another trial (Multi MERCI) used an updated version of the Merci device which showed a higher recanalization (69%) and a lower mortality rate.[42] During that time, another thrombectomy device emerged as an alternative which was called the Penumbra system (Penumbra Inc, Alameda, CA) which prioritized aspiration as the primary mode of thrombectomy (**Fig. 1**B, C). The system consisted of a separator which is passed through the aspiration catheter. The catheter is placed close to the clot under constant aspiration while the

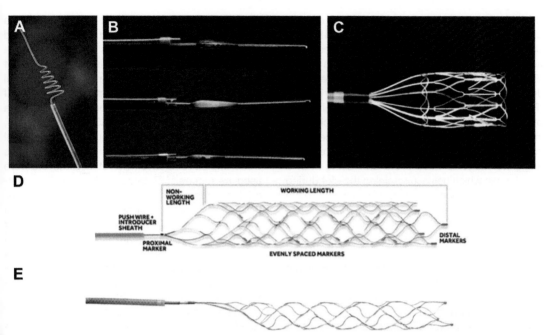

Fig. 1. (*A*) The original Merci device with helicoid loops. (*B,C*) The original Penumbra aspiration system. (D) Solitaire-X stentriever. (*E*). Trevo XP ProVue Stentriever. ([*A-E*] Copyright© Stryker Neurovascular, Reprinted with permission. All Rights Reserved; [*B,C*] Copyright © Penumbra Inc. Reprinted with permission. All Rights Reserved; and [D] Copyright © October 2021 Medtronic, Inc. Reprinted with permission-All Rights Reserved.)

separator is passed to fragment the clot that is aspirated into the catheter. In one of the index trials using the Penumbra system which included 125 patients, successful recanalization was demonstrated in 82% (as compared with 69% with Merci device in Multi-MERCI) although with a similar mortality rate (33%). In the early years, there was a mixed experience with the use of thrombectomy devices. Higher recanalization rates were generally associated with good clinical outcomes and failed recanalization leading to higher complication rates and higher mortality. There was a persistent enthusiasm over improving the design and safety of the devices which led to the emergence of first-generation stent retrievers. The concept of stent retrievers is derived from the success of expandable stents used in the treatment of aneurysms and intracranial atherosclerosis, with the difference being the stents used in thrombectomy are retrievable. The 2 first-generation stent retrievers which received FDA clearance are Solitaire FR (MicroTherapeutic Inc, Irvine, CA) and the Trevo Retriever (Concentric Medical, Mountain View, CA). The SWIFT trial in 2010 conducted a noninferiority trial comparing the Solitaire FR and the Merci Retriever and found a far superior rate of recanalization (TIMI scale 2 or 3) with the Solitaire device (61% vs 24%). A similar noninferiority trial was conducted for the Trevo

device (TREVO 2) which again showed a higher rate of successful recanalization with the Trevo retriever as compared with the Merci Device (86% vs 60%). In 2013, 3 major trials (MR RESCUE, IMS III, and SYNTHESIS) compared MT to medical management for large vessel occlusion, but unfortunately failed to show any benefit of endovascular management. These trials were heavily criticized in the endovascular world because of inconsistencies in patient selection, device selection, and the treatment workflow. Subsequently, in 2015, 5 major trials featured a streamlined treatment algorithm with the use of first-generation stent retrievers instead of Merci device (MR CLEAN, ESCAPE, EXTEND-IA, SWIFT PRIME, REVASCT) which consistently showed a significant benefit of MT in patients with LVO within 6 hours of onset. This finding revolutionized the treatment guidelines for acute ischemic stroke. Over time, there have been constant attempts to improve stent design and delivery mechanisms to improve the first pass recanalization rate with the development of second-generation stent retrievers. Currently, there are many stent retrievers on market with unique mechanical advantages with each. The newer Solitaire- X (Medtronic, Irvine, CA) device offers a unique parametric design that allows dynamic clot integration (**Fig. 1**D. Similarly, the Trevo XP ProVue device offers an open-cell design for softness and optimal clot integration (Stryker, MI, USA) **(Fig. 1E)**. The other stent retrievers include the 3D revascularization device (Penumbra Inc, Alameda, California) **(Fig. 2A)**; Embotrap retrievable stent (Cerenovus/Johnson & Johnson, New Brunswick, New Jersey) **(Fig. 2B)**. The 3D device has a unique architecture of intraluminal chambers to lock and trap clot during the retrieval process. The Embotrap device is similarly uniquely designed to have an outer cage and inner cage to secure the clot along with a distal mesh which helps in retaining the clot during the removal process. All these devices have shown promising results in several recent case series. With a better understanding of clot morphology and their interaction with the vessel wall, there is a great expectation of the development of newer improved, effective, and safe stent retrievers.

Aspiration versus stent

The most common technique during a stent retriever thrombectomy involves the use of aspiration during the retrieval process to provide a negative suction for better grip of the clot in the stent. Additionally, the negative pressure decreases the forward flow to prevent the distal embolization of the disrupted clot. As an alternative to the use of stent, direct aspiration only has been evaluated and used as a technique for thrombectomy. This approach is called the direct aspiration first pass technique (ADAPT) in which a wide bore aspiration catheter is advanced in contact with the clot and a contact aspiration is performed. After 1 or 2 failed attempts, the stent retriever is used as a rescue measure. The advantage of this approach is that it is fast, avoids the manipulation of the vessel with a stent and in addition, more economical if aspiration is successful without the need of a stent. A single-arm ADAPT FAST study, in 2014, used this technique and reported successful revascularization (TICI 2b or 3) in 78% of the cases which improved to 95% when stent retrievers were used as rescue.[43] Subsequently, 2 RCTs evaluated the efficacy of ADAPT technique to the standard stent-retriever first technique. The first trial was the Contact Aspiration versus Stent Retriever for Successful Revascularization (ASTER) which was designed to prove the superiority of the ADAPT technique over the stentreivers.[44] However, the analysis failed to find a significant difference in the rate of successful reperfusion (mTICI score ≥ 2b) between the 2 techniques (83.1% in ADAPT vs 85.4% in stent retriever). Subsequently, the second trial, the COMPASS trial ran a noninferiority study between the 2 techniques whereby the primary endpoint was functional independence at 90 days.[44] The trial observed 90-days independence in 52% of patients with ADAPT as compared with 50% with stent retrievers. Additionally, the rate of successful reperfusion (mTICI score ≥ 2b) was comparable between the 2 techniques (83% in ADAPT and 81% in stent retriever). The study concluded that the ADAPT technique is

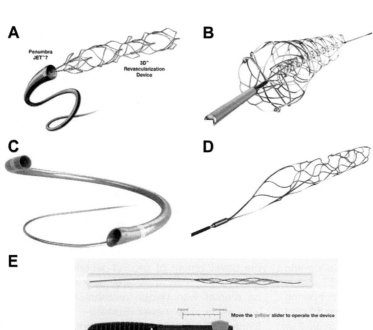

A Penumbra JET™7   3D™ Revascularization Device

B

C

D

E   Expand Compress Move the yellow slider to operate the device

Fig. 2. (A) 3D stentriever (B) Embotrap Stentriever. (C) MIVI Q Catheter System. (D) pRESET stentriever (E) Tigertriever. ([A] Copyright © Penumbra Inc. Reprinted with permission. All Rights Reserved; [B] Copyright © CERENOVUS 2021. Reprinted with permission. All Rights Reserved; [C] Copyright© MIVI Neuroscience, Inc. Reprinted with permission. All Rights Reserved; [D] Copyright © Phenox GmbH, Reprinted with permission. All Rights Reserved; and [E] Image courtesy of Rapid Medial – All rights reserved)

not inferior to stent retrievers to be used as the first pass method for acute large vessel occlusion. Currently, the recommendation from American Heart Association/American Stroke Association does not recommend one technique over the other, but there is a trend among neurointerventionalists to use aspiration as the first pass method for a slightly faster revascularization.[21]

Femoral versus radial versus direct trans-carotid approach

Transfemoral approach has been the traditional method for endovascular access for MT. This is the most common approach the stroke interventionalists is trained to use and often is most comfortable with. Due to time-sensitive nature of the MT, the transfemoral approach is most commonly used. Transradial access is an alternative method of vascular access most commonly adopted in the cardiology world, but has been adopted by neuroendovascular surgeons in a variety of procedures from diagnostic angiograms to aneurysm coiling and carotid stenting. Although difficult femoral access or difficult aortic arch anatomy is the traditional indication for using a transradial approach, it is being used more frequently as a preferred or first-line approach in some centers. The benefits of the transradial approach are multifold and include shorter recovery time, increased patient comfort, lower access site procedural complication rates, and cost savings by avoiding closure devices. However, the radial access is limited by the diameter of the guide catheter that it may allow and may not be suitable in patients with variant arm vascular anatomy or an incomplete palmar arch. The utility of the transradial approach has been recently explored in MT. The need for rapid intravascular access is one of the challenges; therefore, most reports of MT with transradial approach are mostly limited to centers with vast experience with the technique. In a series of 375 patients, Phillips and colleagues compared the transradial access to transfemoral access for MT and found no difference in terms of time to perfusion (median time from imaging to reperfusion 96.5 mins for transfemoral and 95 min for transradial) and clinical outcome (90-days mRS 0–2 of 58% with transfemoral vs 67% with transradial).[45] Additionally, the rate of major access site complication requiring another procedure was higher in transfemoral approach (6.5%) versus none in the transradial approach. Another similar albeit smaller series that included 51 patients found no difference between transradial versus transfemoral approach in terms of single-pass recanalization rate, average number of passes, mean access to reperfusion time, successful revascularization rate, and functional outcomes.[46] Although the transfemoral approach is still the most common access method used in many centers, it is now being more evident that the transradial access could be noninferior to transfemoral approach for MT.

Direct trans-cervical carotid access (TCCA) is also an alternate access route for the anterior circulation and has been infrequently reported for endovascular treatment in strokes. In a reported series of 7 patients, transcarotid puncture was performed after failure of transfemoral access (in 6 patients) and as the initial attempt in one patient (due to tortuosity seen in CT angiogram). Successful revascularization was achieved in all but one patient. One complication of neck hematoma not requiring further surgery was noted.[47] Another report described 6 patients undergoing direct carotid access whereby successful reperfusion was achieved in all patients. One surgical complication involved a neck hematoma that required surgical removal.[48] In a cohort of 7 patients, Scoco and colleagues reported TCCA in 5 patients in which 4 patients achieved $\geq$ TICI 2b reperfusion without any procedural complications.[49] The experience from all these series suggests that direct transcarotid access can be used as a reasonable alternate access when the arch tortuosity or proximal carotid tortuosity is not favorable for transfemoral/transradial access.

Future Directions

Prehospital triage

One of the major challenges in the field is the nonavailability of specific imaging to identify patients with large vessel occlusions who would benefit from rapid intervention and therefore, rely on stroke severity scales which often are unreliable. In this regard, the VIPS device (Volumetric Impedance Phase Shift Spectroscopy, Cerebrotech, California) has been developed by which has the ability to detect LVO based on the difference in the water content in 2 hemispheres. This device is worn by the patient which detects the impendence signals from the hemispheres to see any asymmetry. In a study of 248 patients including patients with acute stroke, other pathologies, and healthy volunteers, the VIPS device was shown to have a sensitivity of 93% and specificity of 92% in detecting LVOs.[50] Similarly, another remarkable development is the SONAS device (BURL Concepts, San Diego, California), a portable, battery-powered ultrasound device for brain perfusion assessment. SONAS works in combination with intravenously injected microbubble contrast agents which are used as signal tracers. Transducers are positioned on both sides of the head to detect hemispheric perfusion deficits (**Fig. 3**A, B). SONAS is CE Mark approved and has been tested clinically for safety and feasibility in patients with stroke.

Improvement of emergency room workflow

Optimization of the emergency room workflow has recently been the prime focus to achieve the shortest door to needle (DTN) and door to groin puncture (DTP) time. One of the key advancements in this regard is the concept and development of a "Neuro ED" which allows a highly coordinated workflow between the ED to the endovascular suite under a highly specialized setup combining the resuscitation bay, imaging, and endovascular suite into one hybrid unit.[51]

Role of artificial intelligence

Machine learning algorithms are being increasingly used to allow a more automated process and reduce lag time in treatment initiation. One of the basic uses is AI-based automated software processing of CT/CTA/CTP imaging to rapidly calculate the ASPECT score, probability of LVO, and the size of penumbra. Another utility of AI is the integration of natural language processing to read the

electronic medical record (Intelligent EMR, iEMR) which allows the extraction of relevant medical history or prior treatment to determine candidacy for thrombolysis/thrombectomy as well as prognostication. With the continued evolution of technology, the scope of AI is expected to be expanded for the rapid formulation of a customized treatment plan for an individual patient.

Endovascular therapy

With rapidly evolving technology and a better understanding of clot morphology and biomechanics, there have been constant improvements in the design and development of stent retrievers. One of the new such concepts is the Lazarus Effect Cover device (Medtronic, Irvine, California) which is a novel nitinol mesh cover that wraps the stentriever during clot retrieval to prevent distal embolism. Similarly, the MIVI-Q Catheter system (MIVI Neurosciences Inc, Prairie, Minnesota) is another innovative aspiration catheter system whereby the proximal portion of the catheter is replaced with a wire, allowing for the increased cross-sectional area to improve the flow rate with aspiration (**Fig. 2**C). Another stent retriever marketed as pRESET 5 to 40 and pRESET LUX (Phenox. Bochum, Germany), currently available in

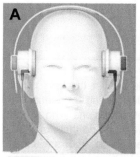
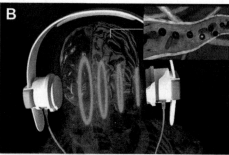
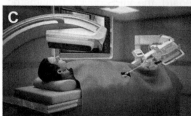
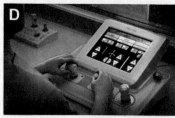
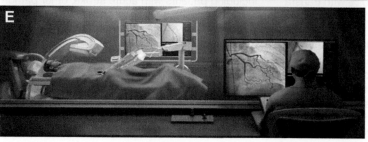

Fig. 3. (*A, B*) SONAS device. Illustration showing the detection of ultrasound waves by the SONAS device after the injection of contrast bubbles (*B*). (*C–E*): Telerobotics CorPath GRX system showing the bedside robotic unit with extended arm(C), The console (*D*), Illustration showing surgeon operating the robotic unit from the console (*E*). ([*A, B*] Copyright © Burl Concepts Inc. Reprinted with permission. All rights reserved; [*C–E*] Copyright © 2021 Corindus, Inc. Reprinted with permission. All Rights Reserved.)

Europe, has a helical slit design to maintain cell shape irrespective of the expansion diameter (**Fig. 2**D). Another innovative design is the radially adjustable stent retriever (Tigertriever, Rapid Medical) which allows the dynamic manipulation of the stent diameter and radial force by the operator with a hand-held slider during the stent deployment (**Fig. 2**E). The primary results of the multicenter TIGER trial have recently been published to show noninferiority of the stent retriever compared with Trevo and Solitaire devices with a first pass successful reperfusion of 57.8% and final successful reperfusion of 95.7%.[52]

Telerobotics in stroke

The use of teleoperated endovascular robots is one of the revolutionary concepts in modern stroke management. Although the concept of robotic MT is relatively new, its utility is now being increasingly realized. The endovascular robot, CorPath GRX system (Corindus, Waltham, MA) initially designed for cardiac angioplasty has now successfully been used in various neuroendovascular procedures including diagnostic angiograms, carotid stenting as well as aneurysm coiling. The robotic system has 3 components including the bedside robotic unit with an extended arm, a single-use cassette with all endovascular supplies, and a remote physician workspace with console (**Fig. 3**C–E). The physician controls the catheter and wire movement at the console outside of the operating room using a joystick, touch screen, and foot pedals. A high-speed local area network allows rapid transmission of the signal to the robotic arm for precise and real-time control of the catheter system without significant time lag. Telerobotics involves the use of robots at one facility which is controlled by an experienced endovascular surgeon at another facility through high-speed fiber network system.[53] The utility of telerobots has been recently tested in an ex vivo proof of concept study whereby robotics endovascular thrombectomy was successfully performed on an artificial human model by an off-site neurosurgeon at a location 5 miles away.[54] With future use in real patients, such a proficient system is likely to complement the existing telestroke system by adding the possibility for intervention at remote locations, thereby considerably optimizing time to treatment.

Summary

We are now in a time when the scope of revolutionizing acute stroke care is enormous, thanks to multi-center collaborations, novel device design, and technological breakthroughs. The field also benefits from robust industry support and generous funding by foundations and government agencies. The last 2 decades have seen rapid and compelling advances in stroke care. With the integration of imaging, pathology, and clinical data into AI platforms, we are not far from the time when acute stroke intervention will be an individualized approach by man and machine to provide the best possible outcome.

CLINICS CARE POINTS

- Mechanical thrombectomy can provide a significant improvement in clinical outcome in stroke patients with large vessel occlusion up to 24 hours from stroke onset
- Optimization of emergency room workflow to achieve shortest door to needle and door to groin puncture time is essential to improve the clinical outcome after stroke therapy
- Both aspiration and stent retriever techniques provide comparable successful reperfusion rate as well as 90 days independence rates after mechanical thrombectomy

DISCLOSURE

The authors have nothing to disclose.

REFERENCES

1. Demaerschalk BM, Berg J, Chong BW, et al. American Telemedicine Association: Telestroke Guidelines. Telemed J E Health 2017;23(5):376–89.
2. Wilcock AD, Schwamm LH, Zubizarreta JR, et al. Reperfusion Treatment and Stroke Outcomes in Hospitals With Telestroke Capacity. JAMA Neurol 2021;78(5):527–35.
3. Kuang H, Najm M, Chakraborty D, et al. Automated ASPECTS on Noncontrast CT Scans in Patients with Acute Ischemic Stroke Using Machine Learning. AJNR Am J Neuroradiol 2019;40(1):33–8.
4. Fassbender K, Walter S, Liu Y, et al. Mobile stroke unit" for hyperacute stroke treatment. Stroke 2003; 34(6):e44.
5. Fassbender K, Grotta JC, Walter S, et al. Mobile stroke units for prehospital thrombolysis, triage, and beyond: benefits and challenges. Lancet Neurol 2017;16(3):227–37.
6. Walter S, Kostopoulos P, Haass A, et al. Diagnosis and treatment of patients with stroke in a mobile stroke unit versus in hospital: a randomised controlled trial. Lancet Neurol 2012;11(5):397–404.

7. Barrett KM, Pizzi MA, Kesari V, et al. Ambulance-based assessment of NIH Stroke Scale with tele-medicine: A feasibility pilot study. J Telemed Telecare 2017;23(4):476–83.

8. Grotta JC, Yamal JM, Parker SA, et al. Prospective, Multicenter, Controlled Trial of Mobile Stroke Units. N Engl J Med 2021;385(11):971–81.

9. Jahan R, Saver JL, Schwamm LH, et al. Association Between Time to Treatment With Endovascular Reperfusion Therapy and Outcomes in Patients With Acute Ischemic Stroke Treated in Clinical Practice. JAMA 2019;322(3):252–63.

10. Bourcier R, Goyal M, Liebeskind DS, et al. Association of Time From Stroke Onset to Groin Puncture With Quality of Reperfusion After Mechanical Thrombectomy: A Meta-analysis of Individual Patient Data From 7 Randomized Clinical Trials. JAMA Neurol 2019;76(4):405–11.

11. Mendez B, Requena M, Aires A, et al. Direct Transfer to Angio-Suite to Reduce Workflow Times and Increase Favorable Clinical Outcome. Stroke 2018; 49(11):2723–7.

12. Goyal M, Menon BK, van Zwam WH, et al. Endovascular thrombectomy after large-vessel ischaemic stroke: a meta-analysis of individual patient data from five randomised trials. Lancet 2016; 387(10029):1723–31.

13. Suzuki K, Matsumaru Y, Takeuchi M, et al. Effect of Mechanical Thrombectomy Without vs With Intravenous Thrombolysis on Functional Outcome Among Patients With Acute Ischemic Stroke: The SKIP Randomized Clinical Trial. JAMA 2021;325(3):244–53.

14. Yang P, Zhang Y, Zhang L, et al. Endovascular Thrombectomy with or without Intravenous Alteplase in Acute Stroke. N Engl J Med 2020;382(21): 1981–93.

15. Zi W, Qiu Z, Li F, et al. Effect of Endovascular Treatment Alone vs Intravenous Alteplase Plus Endovascular Treatment on Functional Independence in Patients With Acute Ischemic Stroke: The DEVT Randomized Clinical Trial. JAMA 2021;325(3): 234–43.

16. Powers WJ, Derdeyn CP, Biller J, et al. 2015 American Heart Association/American Stroke Association Focused Update of the 2013 Guidelines for the Early Management of Patients With Acute Ischemic Stroke Regarding Endovascular Treatment: A Guideline for Healthcare Professionals From the American Heart Association/American Stroke Association. Stroke 2015;46(10):3020–35.

17. Thomalla G, Cheng B, Ebinger M, et al. DWI-FLAIR mismatch for the identification of patients with acute ischaemic stroke within 4.5 h of symptom onset (PRE-FLAIR): a multicentre observational study. Lancet Neurol 2011;10(11):978–86.

18. Nogueira RG, Jadhav AP, Haussen DC, et al. Thrombectomy 6 to 24 Hours after Stroke with a Mismatch between Deficit and Infarct. N Engl J Med 2018; 378(1):11–21.

19. Albers GW, Marks MP, Kemp S, et al. Thrombectomy for Stroke at 6 to 16 Hours with Selection by Perfusion Imaging. N Engl J Med 2018;378(8):708–18.

20. Demaerschalk BM, Scharf EL, Cloft H, et al. Contemporary Management of Acute Ischemic Stroke Across the Continuum: From TeleStroke to Intra-Arterial Management. Mayo Clin Proc 2020;95(7): 1512–29.

21. Powers WJ, Rabinstein AA, Ackerson T, et al. Guidelines for the Early Management of Patients With Acute Ischemic Stroke: 2019 Update to the 2018 Guidelines for the Early Management of Acute Ischemic Stroke: A Guideline for Healthcare Professionals From the American Heart Association/American Stroke Association. Stroke 2019;50(12): e344–418.

22. Christensen S, Mlynash M, Kemp S, et al. Persistent Target Mismatch Profile >24 Hours After Stroke Onset in DEFUSE 3. Stroke 2019;50(3):754–7.

23. Desai SM, Haussen DC, Aghaebrahim A, et al. Thrombectomy 24 hours after stroke: beyond DAWN. J Neurointerv Surg 2018;10(11):1039–42.

24. Bracard S, Ducrocq X, Mas JL, et al. Mechanical thrombectomy after intravenous alteplase versus alteplase alone after stroke (THRACE): a randomised controlled trial. Lancet Neurol 2016;15(11):1138–47.

25. Desilles JP, Consoli A, Redjem H, et al. Successful Reperfusion With Mechanical Thrombectomy Is Associated With Reduced Disability and Mortality in Patients With Pretreatment Diffusion-Weighted Imaging-Alberta Stroke Program Early Computed Tomography Score </=6. Stroke 2017;48(4):963–9.

26. Sarraj A, Hassan AE, Savitz S, et al. Outcomes of Endovascular Thrombectomy vs Medical Management Alone in Patients With Large Ischemic Cores: A Secondary Analysis of the Optimizing Patient's Selection for Endovascular Treatment in Acute Ischemic Stroke (SELECT) Study. JAMA Neurol 2019;76(10):1147–56.

27. Sarraj A, Sangha N, Hussain MS, et al. Endovascular Therapy for Acute Ischemic Stroke With Occlusion of the Middle Cerebral Artery M2 Segment. JAMA Neurol 2016;73(11):1291–6.

28. Saber H, Narayanan S, Palla M, et al. Mechanical thrombectomy for acute ischemic stroke with occlusion of the M2 segment of the middle cerebral artery: a meta-analysis. J Neurointerv Surg 2018; 10(7):620–4.

29. Anadani M, Spiotta A, Alawieh A, et al. Effect of extracranial lesion severity on outcome of endovascular thrombectomy in patients with anterior circulation tandem occlusion: analysis of the TITAN registry. J Neurointerv Surg 2019;11(10):970–4.

30. Haussen DC, Turjman F, Piotin M, et al. Head or Neck First? Speed and Rates of Reperfusion in

Thrombectomy for Tandem Large Vessel Occlusion Strokes. Interv Neurol 2020;8(2–6):92–100.

31. Da Ros V, Scaggiante J, Sallustio F, et al. Carotid Stenting and Mechanical Thrombectomy in Patients with Acute Ischemic Stroke and Tandem Occlusions: Antithrombotic Treatment and Functional Outcome. AJNR Am J Neuroradiol 2020;41(11):2088–93.

32. Zhu F, Hossu G, Soudant M, et al. Effect of emergent carotid stenting during endovascular therapy for acute anterior circulation stroke patients with tandem occlusion: A multicenter, randomized, clinical trial (TITAN) protocol. Int J Stroke 2021;16(3):342–8.

33. Schonewille WJ, Wijman CA, Michel P, et al. Treatment and outcomes of acute basilar artery occlusion in the Basilar Artery International Cooperation Study (BASICS): a prospective registry study. Lancet Neurol 2009;8(8):724–30.

34. Langezaal LCM, van der Hoeven E, Mont'Alverne FJA, et al. Endovascular Therapy for Stroke Due to Basilar-Artery Occlusion. N Engl J Med 2021;384(20): 1910–20.

35. Heldner MR, Zubler C, Mattle HP, et al. National Institutes of Health stroke scale score and vessel occlusion in 2152 patients with acute ischemic stroke. Stroke 2013;44(4):1153–7.

36. Sarraj A, Hassan A, Savitz SI, et al. Endovascular Thrombectomy for Mild Strokes: How Low Should We Go? Stroke 2018;49(10):2398–405.

37. Goyal N, Tsivgoulis G, Malhotra K, et al. Medical Management vs Mechanical Thrombectomy for Mild Strokes: An International Multicenter Study and Systematic Review and Meta-analysis. JAMA Neurol 2020;77(1):16–24.

38. Seners P, Ben Hassen W, Lapergue B, et al. Prediction of Early Neurological Deterioration in Individuals With Minor Stroke and Large Vessel Occlusion Intended for Intravenous Thrombolysis Alone. JAMA Neurol 2021;78(3):321–8.

39. Ravindra VM, Alexander M, Taussky P, et al. Endovascular Thrombectomy for Pediatric Acute Ischemic Stroke: A Multi-Institutional Experience of Technical and Clinical Outcomes. Neurosurgery 2020;88(1):46–54.

40. Al-Mufti F, Schirmer CM, Starke RM, et al. Thrombectomy in special populations: report of the Society of NeuroInterventional Surgery Standards and Guidelines Committee. J Neurointerv Surg 2021. https://doi.org/10.1136/neurintsurg-2021-017888.

41. Smith WS, Sung G, Starkman S, et al. Safety and efficacy of mechanical embolectomy in acute ischemic stroke: results of the MERCI trial. Stroke 2005;36(7):1432–8.

42. Smith WS. Safety of mechanical thrombectomy and intravenous tissue plasminogen activator in acute ischemic stroke. Results of the multi Mechanical Embolus Removal in Cerebral Ischemia (MERCI) trial, part I. AJNR Am J Neuroradiol 2006;27(6): 1177–82.

43. Turk AS, Frei D, Fiorella D, et al. ADAPT FAST study: a direct aspiration first pass technique for acute stroke thrombectomy. J Neurointerv Surg 2014; 6(4):260–4.

44. Lapergue B, Blanc R, Gory B, et al. Effect of Endovascular Contact Aspiration vs Stent Retriever on Revascularization in Patients With Acute Ischemic Stroke and Large Vessel Occlusion: The ASTER Randomized Clinical Trial. JAMA 2017;318(5): 443–52.

45. Phillips TJ, Crockett MT, Selkirk GD, et al. Transradial versus transfemoral access for anterior circulation mechanical thrombectomy: analysis of 375 consecutive cases. Stroke Vasc Neurol 2021;6(2):207–13.

46. Chen SH, Snelling BM, Sur S, et al. Transradial versus transfemoral access for anterior circulation mechanical thrombectomy: comparison of technical and clinical outcomes. J Neurointerv Surg 2019; 11(9):874–8.

47. Jadhav AP, Ribo M, Grandhi R, et al. Transcervical access in acute ischemic stroke. J Neurointerv Surg 2014;6(9):652–7.

48. Wiesmann M, Kalder J, Reich A, et al. Feasibility of combined surgical and endovascular carotid access for interventional treatment of ischemic stroke. J Neurointerv Surg 2016;8(6):571–5.

49. Scoco AN, Addepalli A, Zhu S, et al. Trans-Carotid and Trans-Radial Access for Mechanical Thrombectomy for Acute Ischemic Stroke: A Systematic Review and Meta-Analysis. Cureus 2020;12(6):e8875.

50. Kellner CP, Sauvageau E, Snyder KV, et al. The VITAL study and overall pooled analysis with the VIPS non-invasive stroke detection device. J Neurointerv Surg 2018;10(11):1079–84.

51. Greenberg K, Hedayat HS, Binning MJ, et al. Innovations in Care Delivery of Stroke from Emergency Medical Services to the Neurointerventional Operating Room. Neurosurgery 2019;85(suppl_1): S18–22.

52. Gupta R, Saver JL, Levy E, et al. New Class of Radially Adjustable Stentrievers for Acute Ischemic Stroke: Primary Results of the Multicenter TIGER Trial. Stroke 2021;52(5):1534–44.

53. Panesar SS, Volpi JJ, Lumsden A, et al. Telerobotic stroke intervention: a novel solution to the care dissemination dilemma. J Neurosurg 2019;132(3): 971–8.

54. Singer J, VanOosterhout S, Madder R. Remote robotic endovascular thrombectomy for acute ischaemic stroke. BMJ Neurol Open 2021;3(1):e000141.

Transvenous Embolization Technique for Brain Arteriovenous Malformations

Muhammad Waqas, MBBS[a,b,c], Ammad A. Baig, MD[a,b,c], Elad I. Levy, MD, MBA[a,b,c,d,e,f], Adnan H. Siddiqui, MD, PhD[a,b,c,d,e,f],*

KEYWORDS

- Brain arteriovenous malformation • Rapid ventricular pacing • Transient transvenous pacing
- Transvenous embolization technique

KEY POINTS

- Transvenous embolization is potentially curative for small AVMs with favorable anatomic features, such as inaccessible arterial feeders, deep location, and/or a single draining vein.
- Use of rapid ventricular pacing allows controlled hypotension during embolization. In our experience, the use of pacing in conjunction with temporary balloon occlusion of the feeding artery enhances safe penetration of the nidus with embolizate.
- Complete flow control using temporary balloon occlusion of the arterial feeder, along with the induction of systemic hypotension, is key to successful embolization through the transvenous approach

BACKGROUND

Brain arteriovenous malformations (bAVMs) are characterized by high-flow, abnormal communications between arteries and veins with irregular and fragile plexiform vessels that constitute the nidus.[1] These plexiform vessels are prone to rupture due to an inherent lack of normal smooth-muscle architecture and aberrant angiogenesis causing life-threatening hemorrhage.[2,3] Patients most commonly present with hemorrhage, seizures, headache, or progressive neurologic deficit secondary to a "steal phenomenon" in which blood is carried away from the normal brain tissue.[4–6] The risk of hemorrhage increases after the first hemorrhagic event.[7]

Definitive treatment of a bAVM consists of complete obliteration of the nidus. These lesions vary in size, location, number, and pattern of arterial feeders, as well as the number and location of draining veins. Variation in the angioarchitecture of AVMs makes them among the most challenging intracranial vascular pathologies to treat. Existing modalities for the treatment of bAVMs are microsurgical resection, endovascular embolization, and radiosurgery. These modalities may be used alone or in combination to achieve a cure of the AVM.[8–15]

The role of endovascular embolization is largely regarded as adjunctive to microsurgery or radiosurgery. Curative embolization with a traditional transarterial approach is possible but uncommon.[16] Cure with embolization alone has reported in up to 40% of cases.[16] However, transarterial embolization can help reduce the nidal volume making the lesion amenable to treatment with

a Department of Neurosurgery, Jacobs School of Medicine and Biomedical Sciences, University at Buffalo, Buffalo, NY, USA; b Department of Neurosurgery, Gates Vascular Institute at Kaleida Health, Buffalo, NY, USA; c University at Buffalo Neurosurgery, 100 High Street, Suite B4, Buffalo, NY 14203, USA; d Department of Radiology, Jacobs School of Medicine and Biomedical Sciences, University at Buffalo, Buffalo, NY, USA; e Canon Stroke and Vascular Research Center, University at Buffalo, Buffalo, NY, USA; f Jacobs Institute, Buffalo, NY, USA
* Corresponding author. University at Buffalo Neurosurgery, 100 High Street, Suite B4, Buffalo, NY 14203.
E-mail address: asiddiqui@ubns.com

Neurosurg Clin N Am 33 (2022) 185–191
https://doi.org/10.1016/j.nec.2021.11.001
1042-3680/22/© 2022 Elsevier Inc. All rights reserved.

radiosurgery or can facilitate microsurgical resection.[10–15,17,18] In recent years, transvenous embolization has emerged as an alternative, potentially curative option for bAVMs that are not amenable to transarterial embolization or when other modalities carry unacceptably high risk.

Transvenous embolization was first described for dural arteriovenous fistulas by Halbach and colleagues in 1989.[17] A decade later, Massoud and Hademenos described their model for AVM embolization using transvenous retrograde nidus sclerotherapy under controlled hypotension (TRENSH) technique.[18] The aim of a transvenous approach is better permeation of the embolic agent in the nidus via retrograde flow that is aided by transient arterial flow arrest without risking ischemic complications.[15] In this article, we discuss the current evidence on the utility of transvenous embolization for AVMs. Further, we discuss the technique of transvenous embolization using ventricular pacing.

CURRENT EVIDENCE

As discussed above, transvenous embolization is a relatively new technique. Few centers have published their clinical experience with the use of this technique. A systematic review included 8 studies with 66 patients.[19] The rate of total occlusion was 96.0% and an all-cause mortality rate of 6.0% (95% confidence interval [CI]: 0.0%–11.0%) with no procedure-related death.[19] Procedure-related complications were seen 8.0% of the patients, and additional treatment was required in 6%.[19] However, the safety profile is not uniform across studies. In a prospective study of 21 patients, transvenous embolization was successfully performed in 19 patients.[7] Procedure-related complications were observed in 6 (28.6%) patients, of which 4 were reported to be transient. Complete angiographic obliteration was seen in 16 (84.2%) patients.[7]

The largest single-center case series of transvenous embolization included 51 patients.[20] Three patients developed intracranial hemorrhage (6%), with complete obliteration observed in 49 of 51 patients (96%) after a single embolization session.[20] Most patients (65%) had previously undergone transarterial embolization. Major permanent deficit was seen in only 1 patient.[20]

We previously published our experience of transvenous AVM embolization using adenosine or ventricular pacing to achieve transient cardiac standstill.[21] Embolization was successful in 10 of 12 patients. In 2 patients, the draining vein could not be accessed. Complete obliteration was achieved in 9 of these 10 cases. Two patients experienced intracranial hemorrhage, both of whom made an excellent recovery and achieved functional independence at the 3-month follow-up evaluation.[21]

ILLUSTRATIVE CASE DESCRIPTION
Clinical Presentation

A 16-year-old girl presented with a ruptured right thalamic AVM. The AVM had multiple large feeders predominantly arising from the right posterior cerebral artery (PCA) along with numerous perforating arteries feeding the nidus with a single large vein draining into the straight sinus through the vein of Galen. A ventriculostomy was performed, and the patient was stabilized in the intensive care unit. During the first 3 treatment stages, we performed transarterial embolization of the right PCA feeder with Onyx 38 (ethylene vinyl alcohol copolymer suspended in dimethyl sulfoxide; Medtronic, Dublin, Ireland). No other arterial feeders were large enough for embolization through the transarterial route. Given the small size of the residual nidus, single large draining vein, and lack of another arterial target, we planned transvenous embolization with an intent to achieve a cure. Transvenous embolization of the AVM with concurrent rapid ventricular pacing (RVP) was performed as described later in discussion and in **Fig. 1**.

Technique for Transvenous Embolization

We previously published a detailed description of the principles of the transvenous embolization technique[21] and have provided a summary description here.

Transvenous embolization is performed under general anesthesia. Throughout the procedure, neuromonitoring is conducted via continuous electroencephalography, brainstem auditory evoked responses, and somatosensory evoked potentials. The bilateral femoral region and right neck are prepared and draped in a sterile fashion. A local anesthetic is injected in both groin regions. A 6-French (F) right common femoral artery sheath and a 6F left femoral venous sheath are then inserted using a micropuncture set and modified Seldinger technique; the placement of these sheaths is confirmed fluoroscopically. The right internal jugular vein is accessed under ultrasound guidance, and the 6F venous sheath is advanced under fluoroscopic guidance to the jugular bulb region, along with a 6F Benchmark catheter (Penumbra Inc., Alameda, California). Intravenous heparin (50 U/kg) is then administered to achieve an activated coagulation time (ACT) of greater than 190 seconds.

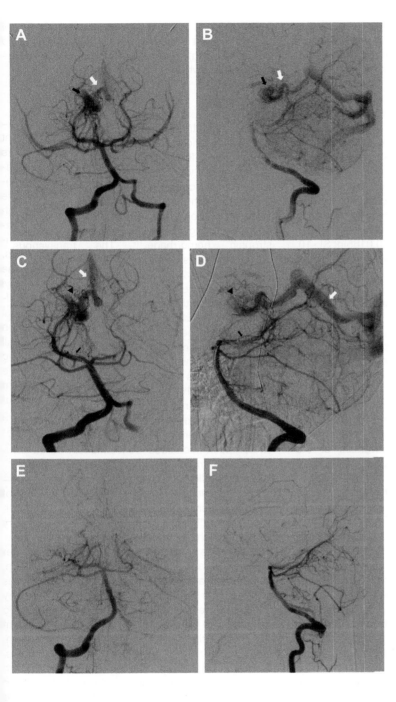

Fig. 1. Right vertebral artery (VA) cranial injection, antero-posterior (AP) (*A*) and lateral (*B*) views, showing right thalamic arteriovenous malformation (AVM) (*black arrows*) with multiple feeders arising from the right posterior cerebral artery (PCA) with a single large vein that drains to the straight sinus (*white arrows*). (*C*) and (*D*), right VA injection, showing the presence of the distal access microcatheter in the straight sinus (*white arrow*). Notice the tip of the Marathon catheter (Medtronic, Dublin, Ireland) wedged into the nidus (*arrowhead*) and the markers of the Scepter balloon (MicroVention-Terumo, Tustin, California) in the right PCA (*black arrows*) to control the inflow of the AVM. Postembolization right VA injection, AP (*E*), and lateral (*F*) views, showing complete obliteration of the nidus.

From the right common femoral artery access, a second 6F Benchmark guide catheter is advanced into the distal cervical internal carotid artery (for anterior circulation lesions) or vertebral artery (for posterior circulation lesions). A Scepter microcatheter balloon (MicroVention-Terumo, Tustin, California) is then parked in the main feeding artery. A cardiac pacer is placed in the right ventricle through 6F femoral venous access.

The 6F Benchmark catheter in the right internal jugular vein is brought up to the right sigmoid sinus and into the right transverse sinus, straight sinus, or superior sagittal sinus, depending on the location of the draining vein. Using a road map of the venous phase of the arterial injection, the target draining vein is catheterized using a Headway Duo microcatheter (MicroVention-Terumo) over a Synchro-2 guidewire (Stryker, Kalamazoo,

Michigan). Arterial injections and roadmaps are repeated as necessary for safe navigation of the target draining vein or veins. For a smaller draining vein, a smaller microcatheter, such as a 0.013in Marathon (Medtronic, Dublin, Ireland), over a 0.010in Synchro 10 wire (Stryker) may be used. The chosen microcatheter is placed in the primary draining vein to enable simultaneous injection of the liquid embolic agent (Onyx 34, Medtronic) into all secondary and tertiary veins. This step ensures that no secondary vein is excluded without adequate penetration of the Onyx 34 into its draining nidus. The blockage of outflow from a draining vein without nidal penetration can lead to hemorrhage. For a large draining vein, a second microcatheter (0.0165in SL-10, Stryker) is placed parallel alongside the more distal microcatheter. This second catheter is kept farther out in the primary draining vein and used to deliver coils and subsequently n-Butyl cyanoacrylate (NBCA) to "jail" the more distal Onyx delivery catheter and for complete occlusion of the draining vein to maximize retrograde Onyx injection into the nidus (referred to as the "reverse pressure cooker technique").[22]

Once the draining vein is satisfactorily catheterized, burst suppression is induced to provide neuroprotection. Cardiac pacing is set at 180 to 200 beats per minute (bpm). Blood pressure is measured to assess the effectiveness of the RVP. For younger patients, higher rates of 220 bpm are used to achieve a sustained arterial pressure of less than 30 mm Hg. The systolic blood pressure (SBP) is lowered to 80 mm Hg. Embolization is performed while the balloon is inflated on the arterial side. During the Onyx injection, burst suppression and hypotension (<90 mm Hg) are maintained.

The principal feeding artery or arteries (basilar, vertebral, internal carotid, middle cerebral, or anterior cerebral) are occluded for <5 min at a time, followed by 2 min of balloon deflation for revascularization before the next balloon inflation. Multiple cycles of RVP are performed during a single inflation with each cycle.

Multiple angiographic runs are used to assess any residual filling. Any residual nidus is aggressively managed with further Onyx embolization. As soon as the venous outflow is obstructed, visualization of the nidus became complicated. Careful assessment of the delayed capillary and venous phases is required to assess residual filling. After a satisfactory embolization result is achieved, the anticoagulation effect is reversed; and all catheters, balloons, and sheaths are removed. If, the Onyx microcatheter remains adherent to the Onyx34 cast, it may be cut at the percutaneous access site of the right internal jugular vein. The patient is kept intubated and hypotensive (SBP 80–90 mm Hg) overnight. SBP parameters are increased slowly by 10 mm Hg per day.

DISCUSSION

The aim of the transvenous approach for bAVMs is better permeation of the embolic agent in the nidus via retrograde flow that is aided by transient arterial flow arrest without risking ischemic complications. A major concern regarding the transvenous approach is the risk of premature occlusion of the vein without nidal penetration, which can lead to the engorgement of the nidus and catastrophic hemorrhage.[15] The transvenous approach is considered when transarterial embolization is not feasible or safe and there is potential to achieve a cure. Current indications for transvenous embolization would include small and compact nidi (<3 cm in diameter), hemorrhagic presentation, deep location, the lack of accessible arterial feeder, and a single draining vein.[15] Recent advancements with flexible microcatheters and microguidewires have improved the safety of the transvenous technique and also helped with better navigation and trackability.[8,23–25]

To achieve deeper, more distal penetration of the embolic agent into the nidus, the transvenous embolization technique conventionally relies on arterial flow arrest either through the use of hypercompliant balloons to generate local hypotension or by attaining systemic hypotension through RVP, adenosine-induced asystole, or hypothermia.[21] The jugular vein is used to establish venous access, and the microcatheter may need to be cut if resistance is encountered during gentle pulling of the catheter at the completion of procedure. We recommend advancing an intermediate catheter closer to the tip of microcatheter to aid in the retrieval of the microcatheter. The use of a microcatheter with a detachable tip may obviate the need to cut the microcatheter at the end of the procedure. An AVM obliteration rate as high as 92.6% has been reported by Mendes and colleagues using this technique.[12] Several other authors have also reported high rates of complete AVM obliteration.[7,13,15]

In cases whereby balloon occlusion is not feasible due to small-sized vessels or high tortuosity, systemic hypotension is a feasible alternative. Using both systemic and local hypotension, Massoud and colleagues achieved improved retrograde nidus contrast filling, deeper embolizate penetration, and decreased intranidal pressure in cases of transvenous embolization.[26,27] Because the intranidal pressure gradient is a major determinant of embolizate permeation and imminent rupture, decreasing this pressure helps curb a major risk of the transvenous technique. Preserving venous outflow is a major concern until complete nidal obliteration is achieved; thus, AVMs with multiple draining veins are best suited for transvenous embolization because the reflux of additional embolizate into accessory draining veins can help prevent premature occlusion.[28] Transient balloon occlusion of arterial feeders is an effective and simple way to achieve local hypotension. For these reasons, transarterial access acts in conjunction with, rather than as an alternative to, the transvenous approach for complete obliteration and better outcomes.

Of the commonly used liquid embolic agents for AVMs, such as NBCA, Onyx, and precipitating hydrophobic injectable liquid (PHIL), Onyx is most suited for transvenous embolization due to its more cohesive and less adhesive properties.[12] These characteristics prevent rapid polymerization of the liquid embolic agent along the vessel wall, allowing it to be injected over long periods of time. This leads to a more controlled and precise embolization, while avoiding immediate and premature occlusion of the draining vein. Compared with arterial embolization, the transvenous injection time for Onyx is shorter, with a decreased interval to the resumption of injection after the formation of the initial plug.[12]

At our center, we have adopted a multidisciplinary approach to transvenous embolization of AVMs with an interventional cardiologist providing transvenous ventricular pacing during embolization. This serves as an adjunct to the temporary balloon occlusion. Transvenous pacing provides superior control of blood pressure compared with pharmacologic agents like adenosine. This requires collaboration with the interventional cardiologist. In our experience, we have not experienced any complications related to RVP, and this technique has previously been applied in cerebrovascular surgery.[29]

SUMMARY

Transvenous embolization is potentially curative for small AVMs with favorable anatomic features, such as inaccessible arterial feeders, deep location, and/or a single draining vein. Successful embolization requires the control of arterial blood flow and successful navigation of the draining vein. This allows the permeation of embolizate into the nidus. Arterial inflow may be controlled using a hypercompliant balloon or systemic hypotension. We have described the use of transvenous RVP and adenosine to achieve transient controlled

hypotension. This requires a multidisciplinary approach, yet provides high chances for complete obliteration of the AVM.

CLINICS CARE POINTS

- Transvenous embolization is potentially curative for small AVMs with favorable anatomic features such as inaccessible arterial feeders, deep location, and/or a single draining vein.
- The use of RVP allows controlled hypotension during embolization. In our experience, the use of pacing in conjunction with temporary balloon occlusion of the feeding artery enhances safe penetration of the nidus with embolizate.
- Complete flow control using temporary balloon occlusion of the arterial feeder, along with the induction of systemic hypotension, is the key to successful embolization through the transvenous approach.

DISCLOSURE

M. Waqas and A.A. Baig—None. E.I. Levy—Consulting fees: Claret Medical, GLG Consulting, Guidepoint Global, Imperial Care, Medtronic, Rebound, StimMed, Misionix, Mosiac, Clarion, IRRAS. Payment or honoraria for lectures, presentations, speakers bureaus, manuscript writing, or educational events: Medtronic; Payment for expert testimony: for rendering medical/legal opinions as an expert. Support for attending meetings and/or travel: Reimbursement for travel and food for some meetings with the CNS and ABNS. Stock or stock options: NeXtGen Biologics, RAPID Medical, Claret Medical, Cognition Medical, Imperative Care, Rebound Therapeutics, StimMed, Three Rivers Medical. A.H. Siddiqui—Consulting fees: Amnis Therapeutics, Apellis Pharmaceuticals, Inc., Boston Scientific, Canon Medical Systems USA, Inc., Cardinal Health 200, LLC, Cerebrotech Medical Systems, Inc., Cerenovus, Cerevatech Medical, Inc., Cordis, Corindus, Inc., Endostream Medical, Ltd, Imperative Care, Integra, IRRAS AB, Medtronic, MicroVention, Minnetronix Neuro, Inc., Penumbra, Q'Apel Medical, Inc., Rapid Medical, Serenity Medical, Inc., Silk Road Medical, StimMed, LLC, Stryker Neurovascular, Three Rivers Medical, Inc., VasSol, Viz.ai, Inc., W.L. Gore & Associates. Leadership or fiduciary role in other board, society, committee, or advocacy group: Secretary of the Board of the Society of Neurointerventional Surgery, Chair of the

Cerebrovascular Section of the AANS/CNS. Stock or stock options: Adona Medical, Inc., Amnis Therapeutics, Bend IT Technologies, Ltd., Blinktbi, Inc., Buffalo Technology Partners, Inc., Cardinal Consultants, LLC, Cerebrotech Medical Systems, Inc., Cerevatech Medical, Inc., Cognition Medical, CVAID Ltd., E8, Inc., Endostream Medical, Ltd, Imperative Care, Inc., Instylla, Inc., International Medical Distribution Partners, Launch NY, Inc., Neuroradial Technologies, Inc., Neurotechnology Investors, Neurovascular Diagnostics, Inc., Perflow Medical, Ltd., Q'Apel Medical, Inc., QAS.ai, Inc., Radical Catheter Technologies, Inc., Rebound Therapeutics Corp. (Purchased 2019 by Integra Lifesciences, Corp), Rist Neurovascular, Inc. (Purchased 2020 by Medtronic), Sense Diagnostics, Inc., Serenity Medical, Inc., Silk Road Medical, Adona Medical, Inc., Amnis Therapeutics, Bend IT Technologies, Ltd., Blinktbi, Inc., Buffalo Technology Partners, Inc., Cardinal Consultants, LLC, Cerebrotech Medical Systems, Inc., Cerevatech Medical, Inc., Cognition Medical, CVAID Ltd., E8, Inc., Endostream Medical, Ltd, Imperative Care, Inc., Instylla, Inc., International Medical Distribution Partners, Launch NY, Inc., Neuroradial Technologies, Inc., Neurotechnology Investors, Neurovascular Diagnostics, Inc., Perflow Medical, Ltd., Q'Apel Medical, Inc., QAS.ai, Inc., Radical Catheter Technologies, Inc., Rebound Therapeutics Corp. (Purchased 2019 by Integra Lifesciences, Corp), Rist Neurovascular, Inc. (Purchased 2020 by Medtronic), Sense Diagnostics, Inc., Serenity Medical, Inc., Silk Road Medical, Songbird Therapy, Spinnaker Medical, Inc., StimMed, LLC, Synchron, Inc., Three Rivers Medical, Inc., Truvic Medical, Inc., Tulavi Therapeutics, Inc., Vastrax, LLC, VICIS, Inc., Viseon, Inc. Other financial or nonfinancial interests: National PI/Steering Committees: Cerenovus EXCELLENT and ARISE II Trial; Medtronic SWIFT PRIME, VANTAGE, EMBOLISE, and SWIFT DIRECT Trials; MicroVention FRED Trial & CONFIDENCE Study; MUSC POSITIVE Trial; Penumbra 3D Separator Trial, COMPASS Trial, INVEST Trial, MIVI neuroscience EVAQ Trial; Rapid Medical SUCCESS Trial; InspireMD C-GUARDIANS IDE Pivotal Trial.

REFERENCES

1. Mouchtouris N, Jabbour PM, Starke RM, et al. Biology of cerebral arteriovenous malformations with a focus on inflammation. J Cereb Blood Flow Metab 2015;35(2):167–75.

2. Winkler EA, Birk H, Burkhardt JK, et al. Reductions in brain pericytes are associated with arteriovenous malformation vascular instability. J Neurosurg 2018;129(6):1464–74.

3. Choudhri O, Ivan ME, Lawton MT. Transvenous approach to intracranial arteriovenous malformations: challenging the axioms of arteriovenous malformation therapy? Neurosurgery 2015;77(4): 644–51 [discussion: 652].

4. Al-Shahi R, Warlow C. A systematic review of the frequency and prognosis of arteriovenous malformations of the brain in adults. Brain 2001;124(Pt 10): 1900–26.

5. Ding D, Starke RM, Kano H, et al. International multicenter cohort study of pediatric brain arteriovenous malformations. Part 1: Predictors of hemorrhagic presentation. J Neurosurg Pediatr 2017;19(2): 127–35.

6. Ding D, Starke RM, Quigg M, et al. Cerebral arteriovenous malformations and epilepsy, Part 1: predictors of seizure presentation. World Neurosurg 2015;84(3):645–52.

7. He Y, Ding Y, Bai W, et al. Safety and efficacy of transvenous embolization of ruptured brain arteriovenous malformations as a last resort: a prospective single-arm study. AJNR Am J Neuroradiol 2019; 40(10):1744–51.

8. Bendok BR, El Tecle NE, El Ahmadieh TY, et al. Advances and innovations in brain arteriovenous malformation surgery. Neurosurgery 2014;74(Suppl 1): S60–73.

9. Hartmann A, Stapf C, Hofmeister C, et al. Determinants of neurological outcome after surgery for brain arteriovenous malformation. Stroke 2000;31(10): 2361–4.

10. van Beijnum J, van der Worp HB, Buis DR, et al. Treatment of brain arteriovenous malformations: a systematic review and meta-analysis. Jama 2011; 306(18):2011–9.

11. Davies JM, Yanamadala V, Lawton MT. Comparative effectiveness of treatments for cerebral arteriovenous malformations: trends in nationwide outcomes from 2000 to 2009. Neurosurg Focus 2012;33(1): E11.

12. Mendes GAC, Kalani MYS, Iosif C, et al. Transvenous curative embolization of cerebral arteriovenous malformations: a prospective cohort study. Neurosurgery 2018;83(5):957–64.

13. Zaki Ghali G, Zaki Ghali MG, Zaki Ghali E. Transvenous embolization of arteriovenous malformations. Clin Neurol Neurosurg 2019;178:70–6.

14. Klurfan P, Gunnarsson T, Haw C, et al. Endovascular treatment of brain arteriovenous malformations: the toronto experience. Interv Neuroradiol 2005;11(1_Suppl):51–6.

15. Chen CJ, Norat P, Ding D, et al. Transvenous embolization of brain arteriovenous malformations: a review of techniques, indications, and outcomes. Neurosurg Focus 2018;45(1):E13.

16. Wu EM, El Ahmadieh TY, McDougall CM, et al. Embolization of brain arteriovenous malformations

with intent to cure: a systematic review. J Neurosurg 2019;132(2):388–99.

17. Halbach VV, Higashida RT, Hieshima GB, et al. Transvenous embolization of dural fistulas involving the cavernous sinus. AJNR Am J Neuroradiol 1989;10(2):377–83.

18. Massoud TF, Hademenos GJ. Transvenous retrograde nidus sclerotherapy under controlled hypotension (TRENSH): a newly proposed treatment for brain arteriovenous malformations–concepts and rationale. Neurosurgery 1999;45(2):351–63 [discussion: 363-355].

19. Fang YB, Byun JS, Liu JM, et al. Transvenous embolization of brain arteriovenous malformations: a systematic review and meta-analysis. J Neurosurg Sci 2019;63(4):468–72.

20. Koyanagi M, Mosimann PJ, Nordmeyer H, et al. The transvenous retrograde pressure cooker technique for the curative embolization of high-grade brain arteriovenous malformations. J Neurointerv Surg 2021;13(7):637–41.

21. Waqas M, Dossani RH, Vakharia K, et al. Complete flow control using transient concurrent rapid ventricular pacing or intravenous adenosine and afferent arterial balloon occlusion during transvenous embolization of cerebral arteriovenous malformations: case series. J Neurointerv Surg 2021;13(4):324–30.

22. Chapot R, Stracke P, Velasco A, et al. The pressure cooker technique for the treatment of brain AVMs. J Neuroradiol 2014;41(1):87–91.

23. Crowley RW, Ducruet AF, McDougall CG, et al. Endovascular advances for brain arteriovenous malformations. Neurosurgery 2014;74(Suppl 1):S74–82.

24. Lv X, Song C, He H, et al. Transvenous retrograde AVM embolization: indications, techniques, complications and outcomes. Interv Neuroradiol 2017; 23(5):504–9.

25. Herial NA, Khan AA, Sherr GT, et al. Detachable-tip microcatheters for liquid embolization of brain arteriovenous malformations and fistulas: a United States Single-Center Experience. Neurosurgery 2015;11(Suppl 3):404–11 [discussion: 411].

26. Massoud TF, Hademenos GJ, Young WL, et al. Can induction of systemic hypotension help prevent nidus rupture complicating arteriovenous malformation embolization?: analysis of underlying mechanism achieved using a theoretical model. AJNR Am J Neuroradiol 2000;21(7):1255–67.

27. Massoud TF. Transvenous retrograde nidus sclerotherapy under controlled hypotension (TRENSH): hemodynamic analysis and concept validation in a pig arteriovenous malformation model. Neurosurgery 2013;73(2):332–42. discussion: 342-333].

28. Hademenos GJ, Massoud TF. Risk of intracranial arteriovenous malformation rupture due to venous drainage impairment. A theoretical analysis. Stroke 1996;27(6):1072–83.

29. Rangel-Castilla L, Russin JJ, Britz GW, et al. Update on transient cardiac standstill in cerebrovascular surgery. Neurosurg Rev 2015;38(4):595–602.

Treatment of Spinal Arteriovenous Malformation and Fistula

Jeff Ehresman, MD[a], Joshua S. Catapano, MD[a], Jacob F. Baranoski, MD[a], Ashutosh P. Jadhav, MD, PhD[b], Andrew F. Ducruet, MD[a], Felipe C. Albuquerque, MD[a],*

KEYWORDS

• Embolization • Endovascular • Fistula • Malformation • Spinal arteriovenous

KEY POINTS

• Endovascular therapy is a highly effective treatment of extradural AVFs, intradural ventral (perimedullary) AVMs, and intramedullary spinal AVMs.

• Incomplete obliteration and recurrence rates of intradural dorsal (dural) AVFs are higher after embolization than after surgical treatment.

• Extradural-intradural (juvenile) and conus medullaris AVMs often require combination treatment, and neurologic improvement rates are poor.

BACKGROUND

Classification and Basic Angioarchitecture

Multiple classification systems have been created to separate spinal arteriovenous malformations (AVMs) based on location, angioarchitecture, and size. The first classification system was created by Di Chiro[1] in 1971 after Di Chiro and colleagues[2] first reported 4 years earlier on the selective angiography of spinal AVMs. Lesions were classified into 3 categories: type I, single-vessel arteriovenous fistula (AVF); type II, glomus AVM; and type II, juvenile AVM. More than 15 years later, in 1987, Di Chiro's group added a fourth type of AVM, those with direct feeders from the anterior spinal artery (ASA).[3] In 2002, Spetzler and colleagues[4] created a schema based on surgical experience that classified the vascular lesions by anatomic locations surrounding or within the spinal cord. This classification is the one primarily used in this review, and it includes (1) extradural AVFs, (2) intradural ventral AVFs, (3) intradural dorsal AVFs, (4) extradural-intradural AVMs, (5) intramedullary AVMs, and (6) conus medullaris AVMs.

Extradural arteriovenous fistulas

Extradural AVFs involve a direct connection between a radicular artery branch and the epidural venous plexus. Venous engorgement or congestion can cause increased retrograde pressure in the medullary veins within the spinal cord, leading to compressive symptoms (**Fig. 1**). Extradural AVFs were further subdivided in 2011 by Rangel-Castilla and colleagues[5] based on whether the radicular artery fed into both the epidural venous plexus and the perimedullary venous plexus (type A) or solely into the epidural venous plexus (type B). Type B extradural AVFs were then further subdivided based on whether the engorged epidural venous plexus compressed the thecal sac (type B1) or did not compress it (type B2).

SUBMISSION CATEGORY: Literature Review

Financial support: None.

[a] Department of Neurosurgery, Barrow Neurological Institute, St. Joseph's Hospital and Medical Center, Phoenix, AZ 85013, USA; [b] Department of Interventional Neurology, Barrow Neurological Institute, St. Joseph's Hospital and Medical Center, Phoenix, AZ, USA

* Corresponding author. c/o Neuroscience Publications, Barrow Neurological Institute, St. Joseph's Hospital and Medical Center, 350 West Thomas Road, Phoenix, AZ 85013.

E-mail address: Neuropub@barrowneuro.org

Neurosurg Clin N Am 33 (2022) 193–206

https://doi.org/10.1016/j.nec.2021.11.005

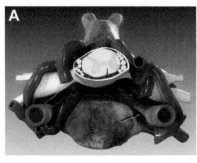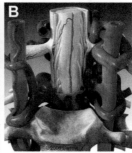

Fig. 1. Extradural arteriovenous fistulas (AVFs). (A) Axial illustration of an extradural AVF along a perforating branch of the left vertebral artery (*arrow*). (B) Illustration of the posterior view of an extradural AVF showing engorgement of the epidural veins, which can produce symptomatic mass effect on adjacent nerve roots and the spinal cord. (*Used with permission from* Barrow Neurological Institute, Phoenix, Arizona.)

Intradural dorsal arteriovenous fistulas

Intradural dorsal AVFs, also known as type I AVMs or spinal dural AVFs, are the most common type of spinal AV shunt.[6] These fistulas are located at the dural nerve root sleeve and involve a radicular feeder artery with a direct connection to a medullary vein (**Fig. 2**).

Intradural ventral arteriovenous fistulas

Intradural ventral AVFs, often referred to as perimedullary type IV AVFs, involve a direct connection between the ASA and the coronal (pial) venous plexus. These AVFs have also been subdivided into the following types: type A, single-feeder with slow flow through the microfistula; type B, multiple feeders with increased flow through a macrofistula; and type C, multiple feeders with fast flow through a giant macrofistula, causing engorgement of the venous plexus (**Fig. 3**).[7]

Extradural-intradural arteriovenous malformations

Extradural-intradural AVMs, otherwise known as type III, juvenile, or metameric AVMs, are often large and complex lesions spanning multiple tissue layers (eg, spinal cord, dura, bone, and skin). These lesions often present in childhood and are associated with various genetic syndromes.[7] Arterial supply often comes from multiple segmental arterial branches. These lesions can drain into any nearby venous plexus (**Fig. 4**).

Intramedullary arteriovenous malformations

Intramedullary AVMs, or type II glomus AVMs, include a classic nidus within the spinal cord and may include multiple arterial branches of the ASA and the posterior spinal artery (PSA) that drain into the coronal venous plexus. These lesions are classified as either compact or diffuse. Intramedullary lesions are often high-flow lesions that are also associated with flow-related aneurysms (**Fig. 5**).[8]

Conus medullaris arteriovenous malformations

Conus medullaris AVMs are complex lesions with multiple direct feeder arteries from the ASA, PSA, and radicular arteries that drain into a complex venous network near the conus medullaris and extend along the cauda equina even to the filum terminale (**Fig. 6**).[9] Rather than existing only as a compact nidus, they are often composed of

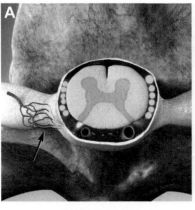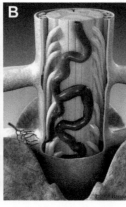

Fig. 2. Intradural dorsal arteriovenous fistulas (AVFs). (A) Axial illustration of an intradural dorsal AVF shows an abnormal radicular feeding artery (*arrow*) along the nerve root on the right. The glomerular network of tiny branches coalesces at the site of the fistula along the dural root sleeve. (B) Posterior view of intradural dorsal AVF shows the dilatation of the coronal venous plexus. In addition to venous outflow obstruction (not shown), arterialization of these veins produces venous hypertension. Focal disruption of the point of the fistula by endovascular or microsurgical methods will obliterate the lesion (*Used with permission from* Barrow Neurological Institute, Phoenix, Arizona.)

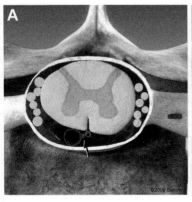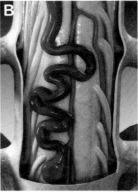

Fig. 3. Intradural ventral arteriovenous fistulas (AVFs). (*A*) Axial illustration of an intradural ventral AVF, a midline lesion derived from a fistulous connection (*arrow*) between the anterior spinal artery and the coronal venous plexus. (*B*) Anterior view of intradural ventral AVF shows the fistula along the anteroinferior aspect of the spinal cord. Proximal and distal to this type A lesion, the course of the anterior spinal artery is normal. (*Used with permission from Barrow Neurological Institute, Phoenix, Arizona.*)

multiple large AVFs that require individual treatment to address the entire lesion.

ENDOVASCULAR TREATMENT AND OUTCOMES
Extradural Arteriovenous Fistulas

Spinal extradural AVFs are unique in that the segmental feeding artery often drains into an epidural venous "pouch"; hence, treatment typically necessitates the embolization of the pouch as well as the feeding artery to prevent AVF recurrence.[10] To achieve this goal, authors of recent case series have used n-butyl cyanoacrylate (NBCA) glue and Onyx (nonadhesive ethylene-vinyl alcohol copolymer dissolved in dimethyl sulfoxide with micronized tantalum powder) as liquid embolisates (**Table 1**).[5,11–16] Although the large sizes of venous pouches and the presence of multiple feeders can impede embolization, most patients achieve positive radiologic and clinical outcomes.[11,15,16] Takai and colleagues[15] evaluated 39 patients who underwent embolization for spinal extradural AVFs, 11 (28%) of whom had either incomplete obliteration or recurrence that was nearly 6 times greater than after surgical treatment. Importantly, however, 8 (72%) of these endovascular patients went on to have neurologic improvement within a median follow-up of 31 months. Similarly, in a study of 20 patients undergoing embolization, Nasr and colleagues[16] found that 19 (95%) of the patients had complete obliteration without recurrence. Both of these studies included the use of either NBCA glue or Onyx and incurred endovascular complication rates of 3% and 10%, respectively.[15,16]

In a 2019 meta-analysis that included 123 treated patients in 11 studies, Byun and colleagues[17] found that most patients were treated solely through endovascular embolization (67.5%) rather than with microsurgery alone

(23.6%) or a combined approach (8.9%). The overall rate of complete obliteration was 83.5%, which did not differ significantly among treatment groups. The overall rate of clinical improvement was 70.7%, which also did not differ among treatment groups. The authors concluded that both endovascular and microsurgical treatments are effective means of treating extradural AVFs.

Intradural Dorsal (Type I) Arteriovenous Fistulas

Intradural dorsal AVFs historically have been treated through surgical ligation of the radicular

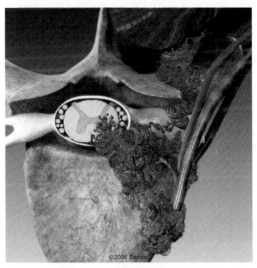

Fig. 4. Extradural-intradural arteriovenous malformations (AVMs). Axial illustration of an extradural-intradural spinal AVM. These treacherous lesions can encompass soft tissues, bone, the spinal canal, the spinal cord, and spinal nerve roots along an entire spinal level. Considerable involvement of multiple structures makes these entities extremely difficult to treat. Although cures have been reported, the primary goal of treatment is usually palliative. (*Used with permission from Barrow Neurological Institute, Phoenix, Arizona.*)

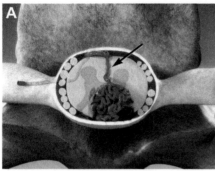
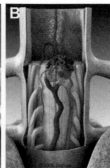

Fig. 5. Intramedullary arteriovenous malformations (AVMs). (A) Axial illustration of a compact intramedullary AVM with an arterial feeder (*arrow*) from the anterior spinal artery identified. Note the discrete, compact mass of the AVM. (B) Posterior view shows additional feeding branches from the posterior spinal artery, which reemphasizes the compact nature of this type of spinal AVM. Portions of the AVM are evident along the surface of the spinal cord. Surgical resection is the mainstay of treatment. Preoperative embolization is reserved for select cases only. (*Used with permission from* Barrow Neurological Institute, Phoenix, Arizona.)

artery feeding the direct connection to a medullary vein.[10] However, the number of published case series detailing the embolization treatment of these lesions has increased in recent years (**Table 2**).[14,18–42] In endovascular treatment, once it has been confirmed (through microcatheter injections) that no normal vessels supplying the spinal cord are distal to the site of the fistula, both the fistula and the proximal intradural draining vein can be embolized.

The combined data from the 3 most recent endovascular series show that postembolization neurologic improvement occurred in 70% of all patients (57/82) despite having overall radiographic treatment failure (incomplete obliteration or recurrence) in 33 (40%) of 82 patients.[14,18,20] Durnford and colleagues[23] compared surgical and endovascular treatments in a cohort of 59 patients (22 embolization, 37 surgery).[23] Complete obliteration was achieved in all 37 patients who underwent surgery compared with only 12 (55%) patients in the endovascular group. In spite of this difference, neurologic outcomes did not differ significantly between the 2 groups. However, in those patients for

whom initial embolization treatment failed, leading to a later surgery, gait scores were significantly worse than in patients who underwent only 1 type of treatment. Because of the low morbidity of endovascular treatment and similar neurologic outcomes between the 2 types of treatment, Durnford and colleagues[23] advocate an initial endovascular attempt; nonetheless, they also recommend a low threshold for conversion to open surgery.

In a 2019 meta-analysis that included 32 studies with a total of 1341 patients undergoing treatment of spinal dural AVF (590 surgery, 751 embolization), surgery was associated with lower proportions of patients with incomplete obliteration and recurrence and higher proportions with a neurologic improvement compared with the corresponding proportions for embolization.[43]

Intradural Ventral (Type IV, Perimedullary) Arteriovenous Malformations

Intradural ventral AVFs are classified into 3 categories. In type A fistulas, the flow between the ASA and the coronal venous plexus is slow, and

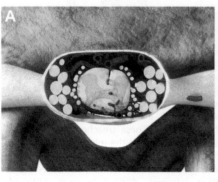
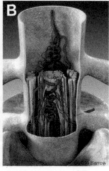

Fig. 6. Conus medullaris arteriovenous malformations (AVMs). (A) Axial illustration of a conus medullaris AVM shows the feeding arteries and draining veins from both the anterior and posterior aspects of the spinal cord. Note the proximity of the AVM to branches of the cauda equina. (B) Posterior view shows the complexity of the angioarchitecture of these lesions. Anterior and posterior spinal arteries, radicular arteries, and anterior and posteriorly draining veins are simultaneously involved. Portions of the AVM can consist of direct AV shunts as well as regions of true AVM nidus. During endovascular treatment, surgical treatment, or both, it is crucial to identify the en passage branches of the anterior and posterior spinal arteries. (*Used with permission from* Barrow Neurological Institute, Phoenix, Arizona.)

Table 1
Case series involving endovascular treatment of spinal extradural arteriovenous fistulas within past 20 y[a]

Study, Y	Endo Tx, No./Total	Embolisate Type (%)	Results, No./Total (%)	Comments
Clarençon et al,[14] 2021	3/15	NBCA (100%) Coils (33%)	Inc. oblit./recurrence: 1/3 (33%) Neuro improvement: 1/2 (50%) Complication rate: 1/3 (33%)	Used pressure cooker technique
Takai et al,[15] 2020	39/280	Coils (6%) NBCA (94%)	Inc. oblit./recurrence: 11/39 (28%) Neuro improvement: 58/81 (72%)[b] Complication rate: 1/39 (3%)	Endo tx associated with higher odds of inc. oblit. than microsurgery (OR 5.7, P = .013)
Kiyosue et al[11] 2017	45/59	NBCA (100%)	Inc. oblit./recurrence: 12/45 (27%) Neuro improvement: 33/51 (65%) Complication rate: 2/45 (4%)	
Nasr et al,[16] 2017	20/24	Onyx (90%) Particle (10%)	Inc. oblit./recurrence: 1/20 (5%) Neuro improvement: 16/20 (80%) Complication rate: 2/20 (10%)	
Ramanthan et al,[12] 2014	3/5	Onyx (100%)	Inc. oblit./recurrence: 1/3 (33%) Neuro improvement: 1/2 (50%) Complication rate: NA	One case used direct percutaneous embo of venous pouch
Rangel-Castilla et al,[5] 2011	7/7	Onyx (100%) NBCA (29%) Coils (14%)	Inc. oblit./recurrence: 0/7 (0%) Neuro improvement: 6/7 (86%) Complication rate: 0/7 (0%)	Divided AVFs into type A, type B1, and type B2
Silva et al,[13] 2007	3/4	Onyx (33%) NBCA (66%) Coils (33%)	Inc. oblit./recurrence: 2/3 (66%) Neuro improvement: 2/3 (66%) Complication rate: 0/3 (0%)	Only included type A spinal extradural AVFs with intradural venous drainage

Abbreviations: AVFs, arteriovenous fistulas; embo, embolization; Endo, endovascular; Inc. oblit., incomplete obliteration; NA, not applicable (studies did not report the variable of interest); Neuro, neurologic; OR, odds ratio; Tx, treatment.
[a] Excludes case reports.
[b] Indicates only value given was from the total cohort due to the lack of stratification.

therefore the ASA often lacks the dilation required for adequate embolization. Type B fistulas are higher-flow lesions with greater ASA dilation and therefore allow for effective embolization of the fistulous site. Type C giant fistulas often lead to large venous networks that can be accessed through transarterial or transvenous routes.[7]

A 2019 case series by Li and colleagues[44] evaluated the effectiveness of embolization in 51 pediatric patients with type B (n = 24) and type C (n = 27) AVFs (**Table 3**).[44–52] The mean age at presentation was 5.6 years and 33 (65%) patients presented with acute neurologic deficits. In patients with low-flow fistulas, the surgeons often used coils or glue alone, whereas a combination was used in high-flow fistulas. Complete obliteration using transarterial embolization occurred in 46 (90%) of the patients, whereas 5 (10%) patients required postembolization microsurgery. Impressively, 42 (82%) of the 51 patients had improved

neurologic scores after embolization. The authors concluded that embolization is a safe and effective means of treating type B and type C macrofistulas.

In line with these results, Phadke and colleagues[46] had previously evaluated perimedullary AVFs in an adult population of 16 endovascularly treated patients and found neurologic improvement in 12 (75%) of 16 patients, with a relatively low rate of incomplete obliteration or recurrence in 4 (25%) of 16 patients at 3-month follow-up. Unlike the 2019 Li and colleagues[44] study, the 2014 Phadke and colleagues[46] study included 10 patients with type A microfistulas and found these AVFs to have greater rates of failed catheterization (4 [40%] vs 1 [10%]) and lower rates of clinical improvement (4 [40%] vs 8 [80%]) than those of macrofistulas. They, therefore, advocate for an initial attempt at embolization, with a low threshold for conversion to microsurgery in patients who have type A AVFs with unfavorable vascular

Table 2
Case series involving endovascular treatment of spinal intradural dorsal (type I) arteriovenous fistulas within past 10 y[a]

Study, Y	Endo Tx, No./Total	Embolisate	Results, No./Total (%)	Comments
Clarençon et al,[14] 2021	12/15	Onyx (27%)[b] NBCA (73%)	Inc. oblit./recurrence: 1/12 (8%) Neuro improvement: 11/12 (92%) Complication rate: 1/12 (8%)	Used pressure cooker technique
Lee HS et al,[18] 2021	56/71	NBCA (100%)	Inc. oblit./recurrence: 27/56 (48%) Neuro improvement: 26/56 (46%) Complication rate: 4/56 (7%)	
Bretonnier et al,[19] 2019	40/63	NA	Inc. oblit./recurrence: 18/40 (45%) Neuro improvement: NA Complication rate: 1/40 (2.5%)	
Kang et al,[20] 2019	14/26	NBCA (100%)	Inc. oblit./recurrence: 5/14 (36%) Neuro improvement: 10/14 (71%) Complication rate: NA	Embo associated with greater risk of recurrence (OR 2.2, P = .046)
Ma et al,[21] 2018	13/94	Onyx (100%)	Inc. oblit./recurrence: 3/13 (23%) Neuro improvement: 9/10 (90%) Complication rate: 0/10 (0%)	
Adrianto et al,[22] 2017	4/9	NBCA (100%)	Inc. oblit./recurrence: 1/4 (25%) Neuro improvement: 2/4 (50%) Complication rate: NA	Study included only patients with concomitant origin of ASA or PSA with sDAVF
Durnford et al,[23] 2017	22/59	NA	Inc. oblit./recurrence: 12/22 (55%) Neuro improvement: 28/57 (49%)[b] Complication rate: 3/22 (14%)	No significant difference in neuro improvement between endo tx and surgery
Lee J et al,[24] 2016	32/37	NA	Inc. oblit./recurrence: 12/32 (38%) Neuro improvement: 24/32 (75%) Complication rate: 0/32 (0%)	
Sasamori et al,[25] 2016	31/50	NBCA (100%)	Inc. oblit./recurrence: 12/31 (39%) Neuro improvement: 33/50 (66%)[b] Complication rate: 4/31 (13%)	
Suh et al,[26] 2016	11/11	NBCA (91%) Onyx (9%)	Inc. oblit./recurrence: 1/10 (10%) Neuro improvement: 9/11 (82%) Complication rate: 0/11 (0%)	Used "induced-wedge technique" by blocking blood flow at the proximal portion of microcatheter during embo
Zogopoulos et al,[27] 2016	10/14	NBCA (80%) Coils (60%)	Inc. oblit./recurrence: 1/10 (10%) Neuro improvement: 4/10 (40%) Complication rate: 1/10 (10%)	

(continued on next page)

Table 2
(continued)

Study, Y	Endo Tx, No./Total	Embolisate	Results, No./Total (%)	Comments
Chibbaro et al,[28] 2015	120/142	NA	Inc. oblit./recurrence: 8/120 (7%) Neuro improvement: NA Complication rate: 0/120 (0%)	
Ozkan et al,[29] 2015	5/30	NBCA (100%)	Inc. oblit./recurrence: 2/5 (40%) Neuro improvement: NA Complication rate: 0/5 (0%)	
Shin et al,[30] 2015	9/15	NBCA (100%)	Inc. oblit./recurrence: 13/15 (87%)[b] Neuro improvement: 6/9 (67%) Complication rate: 1/9 (11%)	
Gokhale et al,[31] 2014	10/27	Onyx (50%) NBCA (50%)	Inc. oblit./recurrence: 3/10 (30%) Neuro improvement: NA Complication rate: 1/10 (10%)	
Qi et al,[32] 2014	12/52	NBCA (100%)	Inc. oblit./recurrence: 8/12 (67%) Neuro improvement: NA Complication rate: 0/12 (0%)	
Tsuruta et al,[33] 2014	98/98	NBCA (78%) Coil (27%)	Inc. oblit./recurrence: 10/98 (10%) Neuro improvement: 49/98 (50%) Complication rate: 3/98 (3%)	
Cho et al,[34] 2013	26/32	NBCA (100%)	Inc. oblit./recurrence: 4/26 (15%) Neuro improvement: 8/26 (31%) Complication rate: 5/26 (19%)	
Gemmete et al,[35] 2013	29/33	Onyx (31%) NBCA (69%)	Inc. oblit./recurrence: 5/29 (17%) Neuro improvement: NA Complication rate: 1/29 (3%)	
Inagawa et al,[36] 2013	12/14	NBCA (100%)	Inc. oblit./recurrence: 5/12 (42%) Neuro improvement: 5/12 (42%) Complication rate: 2/12 (17%)	
Kirsch et al,[37] 2013	61/78	NBCA (100%)	Inc. oblit./recurrence: 14/61 (23%) Neuro improvement: 53/72 (74%)[b] Complication rate: 1/61 (2%)	
Su et al,[38] 2013	40/40	NBCA (100%)	Inc. oblit./recurrence: 16/40 (40%) Neuro improvement: NA Complication rate: 2/40 (5%)	

(continued on next page)

Table 2
(continued)

Study, Y	Endo Tx, No./Total	Embolisate	Results, No./Total (%)	Comments
Takai et al,[39] 2013	5/27	NA	Inc. oblit./recurrence: 0/5 (0%) Neuro improvement: 3/5 (60%) Complication rate: 0/5 (0%)	
Cenzato et al,[40] 2012	10/65	NBCA (100%)	Inc. oblit./recurrence: 3/10 (30%) Neuro improvement: NA Complication rate: 0/10 (0%)	
Wakao et al,[41] 2012	14/30	NBCA (100%)	Inc. oblit./recurrence: NA Neuro improvement: 7/14 (50%) Complication rate: 0/14 (0%)	
Ruiz-Juretschke et al,[42] 2011	9/19	NBCA (100%)	Inc. oblit./recurrence: 4/9 (44%) Neuro improvement: 5/9 (56%) Complication rate: 1/9 (11%)	

Abbreviations: ASA, anterior spinal artery; Embo, embolization; Endo, endovascular; Inc. oblit., incomplete obliteration; NA, not applicable (studies did not report the variable of interest); NBCA, n-butyl-cyanoacrylate; Neuro, neurologic; OR, odds ratio; PSA, posterior spinal artery; sDAVF, spinal dural arteriovenous fistula; Tx, treatment.
   [a] Excludes case reports.
   [b] Indicates only value given was from the total cohort due to the lack of stratification.

architecture. In a 2013 pooled analysis of 28 studies that included 213 patients with all 3 subtypes of intradural ventral AVMs, Gross and Du[53] found the endovascular obliteration rate to be 74% with a 75% rate of neurologic improvement. They concluded that the results of their analysis confirmed the effectiveness of endovascular therapy for these lesions.

Extradural–Intradural (Type III, Juvenile, Metameric) Arteriovenous Fistulas

The literature detailing treatments of extradural–intradural AVMs is scarce, both because of the rarity of the lesions and because of the considerable difficulty in treating them. The treatment of these lesions often requires multiple stages and involves a combination of coils, liquid embolic agents, and surgical resection.[9]

Kalani and colleagues[54] reported 2 cases of endovascular treatment of pediatric spinal AVMs in which both patients presented with paraparesis. One patient underwent transarterial embolization exclusively, and 1 patient underwent both embolization and microsurgery (**Table 4**).[54,55] Although the first patient experienced a procedure-related subarachnoid hemorrhage and was lost to follow-up, the second patient experienced no

complications and had substantially improved neurologic function at last follow-up, 2 months after the procedure. Alomari and colleagues[55] also presented the cases of 2 pediatric patients with extradural–intradural AVMs who underwent embolization and surgery without neurologic improvement because of the continuing growth of lesions. These reports demonstrate the vast complexity and difficulty in treating these lesions, and their findings indicate that treatments are often high risk, with the progression of the disease likely to lead to debilitating outcomes.

Intramedullary (Type II, Glomus) Arteriovenous Fistulas

Similar to the management of intradural dorsal AVFs, the treatment of intramedullary AVMs has historically been surgical resection as the treatment of choice.[7] However, patients who are selected for endovascular treatment because of favorable angioarchitecture may have favorable neurologic outcomes (**Table 5**).[47,56,57] In 2012, Lv and colleagues[47] reported on their use of Onyx to embolize intramedullary AVMs in 7 adult patients, and although the rate of incomplete obliteration or radiographic recurrence was relatively high (3 [43%] of 7 patients), neurologic

Table 3
Case series involving endovascular treatment of spinal intradural ventral (perimedullary) arteriovenous fistulas within past 20 y[a]

Study, Y	Endo Tx, No./Total	Embolisate	Results, No./Total (%)	Comments
Li et al,[44] 2019	51/51	NBCA (100%) Coils (100%)	Inc. oblit./recurrence: 5/51 (10%) Neuro improvement: 42/51 (82%) Complication rate: 1/51 (2%)	Type B: n = 24 Type C: n = 27 Pediatric population
Cho et al,[45] 2016	5/10	Onyx (NA) NBCA (NA) Coils (NA)	Inc. oblit./recurrence: 3/5 (60%) Neuro improvement: 4/5 (80%) Complication rate: 0/5 (0%)	Type B: n = 2 Type C: n = 3
Phadke et al,[46] 2014	16/21	NBCA (100%)	Inc. oblit./recurrence: 4/16 (25%) Neuro improvement: 12/16 (75%) Complication rate: 1/16 (6%)	Type A: n = 5 Type B: n = 9 Type C: n = 2
Lv et al,[47] 2012	4/11	Onyx (50%) Coils (100%)	Inc. oblit./recurrence: 1/4 (25%) Neuro improvement: NA Complication rate: 0/4 (0%)	
Casasco et al,[48] 2011	2/2	Onyx (50%) NBCA (50%) Coils (100%)	Inc. oblit./recurrence: 2/2 (100%) Neuro improvement: 2/2 (100%) Complication rate: 0/2 (0%)	Used direct percutaneous venous puncture for embo
Meng et al,[49] 2010	19/19	NA	Inc. oblit./recurrence: 6/19 (32%) Neuro improvement: 15/19 (79%) Complication rate: NA	Pediatric population
Cho et al,[50] 2005	11/19	NA	Inc. oblit./recurrence: 6/11 (55%) Neuro improvement: 5/11 (45%) Complication rate: NA	Type A: n = 5 Type B: n = 2 Type C: n = 4
Oran et al,[51] 2005	5/5	NBCA (100%)	Inc. oblit./recurrence: 1/5 (20%) Neuro improvement: 5/5 (100%) Complication rate: 0/5 (0%)	Type A: n = 5
Rodesch et al,[52] 2005	18/32	NBCA (100%)	Inc. oblit./recurrence: 6/18 (33%) Neuro improvement: 18/18 (100%) Complication rate: 7/32 (22%)[b]	Separated into macrofistulas (n = 7) and microfistulas (n = 25)

Abbreviations: Embo, embolization; Endo, endovascular; Inc. oblit., incomplete obliteration; NA, not applicable (studies did not report the variable of interest); NBCA, n-butyl-cyanoacrylate; Neuro, neurologic; Tx, treatment.
[a] Excludes case reports.
[b] Indicates only value given was from the total cohort due to the lack of stratification.

Table 4
Case series involving endovascular treatment of spinal extradural-intradural (type III, juvenile, or metameric) arteriovenous malformations within past 20 y[a]

Study, Y	Endo Tx, No./Total	Embolisate	Results, No./Total (%)	Comments
Kalani et al,[54] 2012	2/9	Onyx (100%)	Inc. oblit./recurrence: 2/2 (100%) Neuro improvement: 2/2 (100%) Complication rate: 1/2 (50%)	Klippel–Trénaunay–Weber syndrome (n = 4) HHT syndrome (n = 1)
Alomari et al,[55] 2011	2/6	NA	Inc. oblit./recurrence: 0/1 (0%) Neuro improvement: 0/1 (0%) Complication rate: NA	Pediatric population with CLOVES syndrome

Abbreviations: CLOVES, congenital lipomatous overgrowth; vascular malformations, epidermal nevi; and scoliosis/skeletal/spinal anomalies; Endo, endovascular; HHT, hereditary hemorrhagic telangiectasia; Inc. oblit., incomplete obliteration; NA, not applicable (studies did not report the variable of interest); Neuro, neurologic; Tx, treatment.
[a] Excludes case reports.

improvement occurred in 5 patients (71%) and 1 patient remained asymptomatic. Similarly, Corkill and colleagues[56] reported in 2007 that 17 patients who underwent Onyx embolization for intramedullary AVMs had a relatively high rate of incomplete obliteration or radiographic recurrence (10 [59%] of 17); however, they had a high rate of neurologic improvement (14 [82%] of 17) at a mean follow-up of 2 years. These results are in line with those of a 2013 pooled meta-analysis by Gross and Du,[58] who found that despite an overall rate of complete obliteration with endovascular treatment of only 33%, even partial obliteration substantially decreased the rate of future hemorrhage and neurologic decline. Therefore, by emphasizing proper patient selection, these series demonstrate embolization to be a highly effective treatment of these lesions that have historically been treated surgically.

Table 5
Case series involving endovascular treatment of spinal intramedullary (type II, glomus) arteriovenous malformations within past 20 y[a]

Author, Y[Ref.]	Endo Tx, No./Total	Embolisate	Results, No./Total (%)	Comments
Lv et al,[47] 2012	7/11	Onyx (100%)	Inc. oblit./recurrence: 3/7 (43%) Neuro improvement: 5/7 (71%) Complication rate: 1/7 (14%)	
Corkill et al,[56] 2007	17/17	Onyx (100%)	Inc. oblit./recurrence: 10/17 (59%) Neuro improvement: 14/17 (82%) Complication rate: 2/17 (12%)	
Cullen et al,[57] 2006	9/13	NBCA (100%)	Inc. oblit./recurrence: 2/9 (22%) Neuro improvement: NA Complication rate: 1/9 (11%)	Pediatric population; all patients presented younger than 2 y of age

Abbreviations: Endo, endovascular; Inc. oblit., incomplete obliteration; NA, not applicable (studies did not report the variable of interest); NBCA, n-butyl-cyanoacrylate; Neuro, neurologic; Tx, treatment.
[a] Excludes case reports.

Conus Medullaris Arteriovenous Malformations

Conus medullaris AVMs are difficult-to-treat lesions because they often have multiple direct shunts feeding a complex venous network at the conus.[7] Their management usually involves both embolization and microsurgical resection. Kalani and colleagues[54] described the course of 3 pediatric patients who underwent transarterial embolization (n = 3) and surgery (n = 2) for conus AVMs (**Table 6**).[54,59] In the 3 endovascularly treated patients, 2 were found to have no residual AVM at 1-month follow-up. The third patient was followed up for more than 3 years and was found to have significantly improved neurologic function, despite eventual asymptomatic radiographic recurrence.

In the largest case series to date, Wilson and colleagues[59] described 8 patients in 2012 who underwent embolization prior to microsurgery. Treatment led to complete obliteration of the AVM in 7 (88%) of 8 patients, and 3 (43%) of 7 patients with follow-up had neurologic improvement at a mean follow-up of 70 months. Because these lesions often involve multiple large AVFs, such studies demonstrate that multimodality endovascular treatment (eg, coils, glue, Onyx) and surgical resection are often required. Although conus medullaris AVMs are difficult to treat, neurologic outcomes can nonetheless be improved with these multidisciplinary interventions.[54,59]

DISCUSSION
NBCA Versus Onyx

The goal when using any embolization agent is to allow for a highly selective, controlled release to fill the entire volume of the targeted vessels.

NBCA, an acrylic glue, has been the most commonly preferred material for neurointerventionalists. Previously, the preferred embolization agent was polyvinyl alcohol particles, which adhere to vessel walls and clot blood through physical aggregation.[10] However, the recanalization rate after the use of polyvinyl alcohol in spinal AVMs is nearly 80%.[10] NBCA ("glue"), therefore, became the preferred material because of its ease of use and lower recanalization rate. As an acrylic glue, NBCA polymerizes when it comes into contact with blood, and it is radiopaque when mixed with tantalum powder. However, one issue with NBCA glue is that it can adhere the microcatheter to the vessel when the microcatheter is left in the vessel too long during embolization. Most recently, Onyx, a more viscous mixture of ethylene-vinyl alcohol and micronized tantalum powder suspended in dimethyl sulfoxide, has come into widespread use. Rather than functioning through physical aggregation or polymerization, Onyx works by precipitating in the vessel after the dimethyl sulfoxide diffuses out of the vessel.[60] Much of the rapid adoption of Onyx in the treatment of spinal AVMs has occurred because it provides improved operator control and produces impressive rates of curative therapy in cerebral AVMs.

There are no recent direct randomized controlled comparisons of NBCA and Onyx in terms of complete obliteration, recanalization, and complications in the treatment of spinal AVMs. However, in a 2019 meta-analysis of surgical versus endovascular treatment of intradural dorsal AVFs, Goyal and colleagues[43] determined that Onyx was associated with significantly higher odds of incomplete obliteration and recanalization

Table 6
Case series involving endovascular treatment of spinal arteriovenous malformations at the conus within past 20 y[a]

Author, Y[Ref.]	Endo Tx, No./Total	Embolisate	Results, No./Total (%)	Comments
Wilson et al,[59] 2012	8/16	Onyx or NBCA (% NA)	Inc. oblit./recurrence: 1/8 (12%) Neuro improvement: 3/7 (43%) Complication rate: 0/8 (0%)	Embo was followed by microsurgical resection
Kalani et al,[54] 2012	3/9	NA	Inc. oblit./recurrence: 1/3 (33%) Neuro improvement: 1/3 (33%) Complication rate: 1/3 (33%)	Pediatric population

Abbreviations: Embo, embolization; Endo, endovascular; Inc. oblit., incomplete obliteration; NA, not applicable (studies did not report the variable of interest); NBCA, n-butyl-cyanoacrylate; Neuro, neurologic; Tx, treatment.
[a] Excludes case reports.

compared with NBCA. Blackburn and colleagues[61] had posited in 2014 that the incomplete obliteration and recanalization with Onyx may be due in part to the higher viscosity of Onyx limiting penetration into the draining vein, which is critical to preventing recanalization. However, as early as 2010, Loh and colleagues,[60] reporting on the Onyx Trial that started in 2001, noted that Onyx demonstrated considerably better radiographic outcomes than NBCA with its increased use in treating brain AVMs over the years. Therefore, it is possible for the rates of initial success with Onyx to improve over time as learning curves flatten and operator techniques improve.

SUMMARY

The rapid pace of innovations in the realms of endovascular techniques and devices continues to move the field toward broader indications and improved patient outcomes. Although much of the treatment success for spinal AVMs remains dependent on the type of lesion, endovascular therapies are becoming increasingly effective as both primary and adjunct therapies.

CLINICS CARE POINTS

- Extradural AVF: Endovascular treatment, compared with surgery, has similar rates of complete obliteration and neurologic improvement.

- Intradural dorsal AVF: Surgery has been demonstrated to have high rates of complete obliteration, although neurologic improvement is equivocal between surgery and endovascular treatment.

- Intradural ventral AVM: Endovascular treatment of low-flow type A lesions poses technical challenges, but endovascular treatment of type B and type C lesions has been demonstrated to be highly effective.

- Extradural-intradural AVM: Regardless of the type of treatment of these complex lesions, the disease often progresses to a debilitating outcome.

- Intramedullary AVM: Complete obliteration rates are low with endovascular treatment; however, neurologic improvement rates are high, even with only partial obliteration.

- Conus medullaris AVM: Combination therapy is often required for these AVMs, resulting in high complete obliteration rates but relatively low rates of neurologic improvement.

ACKNOWLEDGMENTS

The authors thank the staff of Neuroscience Publications at Barrow Neurologic Institute for assistance with manuscript preparation.

DISCLOSURE

The authors have no personal, financial, or institutional interest in any of the drugs, materials, or devices described in this article.

REFERENCES

1. Di Chiro G. Angiography of obstructive vascular disease of the spinal cord. Radiology 1971;100(3): 607–14.
2. Di Chiro G, Doppman J, Ommaya AK. Selective arteriography of arteriovenous aneurysms of spinal cord. Radiology 1967;88(6):1065–77.
3. Rosenblum B, Oldfield EH, Doppman JL, et al. Spinal arteriovenous malformations: a comparison of dural arteriovenous fistulas and intradural AVM's in 81 patients. J Neurosurg 1987;67(6):795–802.
4. Spetzler RF, Detwiler PW, Riina HA, et al. Modified classification of spinal cord vascular lesions. J Neurosurg 2002;96(2 Suppl):145–56.
5. Rangel-Castilla L, Holman PJ, Krishna C, et al. Spinal extradural arteriovenous fistulas: a clinical and radiological description of different types and their novel treatment with Onyx. J Neurosurg Spine 2011;15(5):541–9.
6. Takai K. Spinal arteriovenous shunts: angioarchitecture and historical changes in classification. Neurol Med Chir (Tokyo) 2017;57(7):356–65.
7. Ducruet AF, Crowley RW, McDougall CG, et al. Endovascular management of spinal arteriovenous malformations. J Neurointerv Surg 2013;5(6): 605–11.
8. Rangel-Castilla L, Russin JJ, Zaidi HA, et al. Contemporary management of spinal AVFs and AVMs: lessons learned from 110 cases. Neurosurg Focus 2014;37(3):E14.
9. Niimi Y, Uchiyama N, Elijovich L, et al. Spinal arteriovenous metameric syndrome: clinical manifestations and endovascular management. AJNR Am J Neuroradiol 2013;34(2):457–63.
10. Brinjikji W, Lanzino G. Endovascular treatment of spinal arteriovenous malformations. Handb Clin Neurol 2017;143:161–74.
11. Kiyosue H, Matsumaru Y, Niimi Y, et al. Angiographic and clinical characteristics of thoracolumbar spinal epidural and dural arteriovenous fistulas. Stroke 2017;48(12):3215–22.
12. Ramanathan D, Levitt MR, Sekhar LN, et al. Management of spinal epidural arteriovenous fistulas: interventional techniques and results. J Neurointerv Surg 2014;6(2):144–9.

13. Silva N Jr, Januel AC, Tall P, et al. Spinal epidural arteriovenous fistulas associated with progressive myelopathy. Report of four cases. J Neurosurg Spine 2007;6(6):552–8.

14. Clarencon F, Stracke CP, Shotar E, et al. Pressure cooker technique for endovascular treatment of spinal arteriovenous fistulas: experience in 15 cases. AJNR Am J Neuroradiol 2021;42(7):1270–5.

15. Takai K, Endo T, Yasuhara T, et al. Microsurgical versus endovascular treatment of spinal epidural arteriovenous fistulas with intradural venous drainage: a multicenter study of 81 patients. J Neurosurg Spine 2020;24:1–11.

16. Nasr DM, Brinjikji W, Clarke MJ, et al. Clinical presentation and treatment outcomes of spinal epidural arteriovenous fistulas. J Neurosurg Spine 2017; 26(5):613–20.

17. Byun JS, Tsang ACO, Hilditch CA, et al. Presentation and outcomes of patients with thoracic and lumbosacral spinal epidural arteriovenous fistulas: a systematic review and meta-analysis. J Neurointerv Surg 2019;11(1):95–8.

18. Lee HS, Kang HS, Kim SM, et al. Treatment strategy to maximize the treatment outcome of spinal dural arteriovenous fistula after initial endovascular embolization attempt at diagnostic angiography. Sci Rep 2021;11(1):10004.

19. Bretonnier M, Henaux PL, Gaberel T, et al. Spinal dural arteriovenous fistulas: clinical outcome after surgery versus embolization: a retrospective study. World Neurosurg 2019;127:e943–9.

20. Kang MS, Kim KH, Park JY, et al. Comparison of endovascular embolization and surgery in the treatment of spinal intradural dorsal arteriovenous fistulas. World Neurosurg 2019;122:e1519–27.

21. Ma Y, Chen S, Peng C, et al. Clinical outcomes and prognostic factors in patients with spinal dural arteriovenous fistulas: a prospective cohort study in two Chinese centres. BMJ Open 2018;8(1):e019800.

22. Adrianto Y, Yang KH, Koo HW, et al. Concomitant origin of the anterior or posterior spinal artery with the feeder of a spinal dural arteriovenous fistula (SDAVF). J Neurointerv Surg 2017;9(4):405–10.

23. Durnford AJ, Hempenstall J, Sadek AR, et al. Degree and duration of functional improvement on long-term follow-up of spinal dural arteriovenous fistulae occluded by endovascular and surgical treatment. World Neurosurg 2017;107:488–94.

24. Lee J, Lim YM, Suh DC, et al. Clinical presentation, imaging findings, and prognosis of spinal dural arteriovenous fistula. J Clin Neurosci 2016;26:105–9.

25. Sasamori T, Hida K, Yano S, et al. Long-term outcomes after surgical and endovascular treatment of spinal dural arteriovenous fistulae. Eur Spine J 2016;25(3):748–54.

26. Suh DC, Cho SH, Park JE, et al. Induced-wedge technique to improve liquid embolic agent penetration into spinal dural arteriovenous fistula. World Neurosurg 2016;96:309–15.

27. Zogopoulos P, Nakamura H, Ozaki T, et al. Endovascular and surgical treatment of spinal dural arteriovenous fistulas: assessment of post-treatment clinical outcome. Neurol Med Chir (Tokyo) 2016;56(1):27–32.

28. Chibbaro S, Gory B, Marsella M, et al. Surgical management of spinal dural arteriovenous fistulas. J Clin Neurosci 2015;22(1):180–3.

29. Ozkan N, Kreitschmann-Andermahr I, Goerike SL, et al. Single center experience with treatment of spinal dural arteriovenous fistulas. Neurosurg Rev 2015;38(4):683–92.

30. Shin DA, Park KY, Ji GY, et al. The use of magnetic resonance imaging in predicting the clinical outcome of spinal arteriovenous fistula. Yonsei Med J 2015;56(2):397–402.

31. Gokhale S, Khan SA, McDonagh DL, et al. Comparison of surgical and endovascular approach in management of spinal dural arteriovenous fistulas: a single center experience of 27 patients. Surg Neurol Int 2014;5:7.

32. Qi X, Lv L, Han K, et al. Analysis of the embolization spinal dural arteriovenous fistula and surgical treatments on 52 cases of the patients. Int J Clin Exp Med 2014;7(9):3062–71.

33. Tsuruta W, Matsumaru Y, Miyachi S, et al. Endovascular treatment of spinal vascular lesion in Japan: Japanese Registry of Neuroendovascular Therapy (JR-NET) and JR-NET2. Neurol Med Chir (Tokyo) 2014;54(1):72–8.

34. Cho WS, Kim KJ, Kwon OK, et al. Clinical features and treatment outcomes of the spinal arteriovenous fistulas and malformation: clinical article. J Neurosurg Spine 2013;19(2):207–16.

35. Gemmete JJ, Chaudhary N, Elias AE, et al. Spinal dural arteriovenous fistulas: clinical experience with endovascular treatment as a primary therapy at 2 academic referral centers. AJNR Am J Neuroradiol 2013;34(10):1974–9.

36. Inagawa S, Yamashita S, Hiramatsu H, et al. Clinical results after the multidisciplinary treatment of spinal arteriovenous fistulas. Jpn J Radiol 2013;31(7):455–64.

37. Kirsch M, Berg-Dammer E, Musahl C, et al. Endovascular management of spinal dural arteriovenous fistulas in 78 patients. Neuroradiology 2013;55(3):337–43.

38. Su IC, terBrugge KG, Willinsky RA, et al. Factors determining the success of endovascular treatments among patients with spinal dural arteriovenous fistulas. Neuroradiology 2013;55(11):1389–95.

39. Takai K, Kin T, Oyama H, et al. Three-dimensional angioarchitecture of spinal dural arteriovenous fistulas, with special reference to the intradural retrograde venous drainage system. J Neurosurg Spine 2013;18(4):398–408.

40. Cenzato M, Debernardi A, Stefini R, et al. Spinal dural arteriovenous fistulas: outcome and prognostic factors. Neurosurg Focus 2012;32(5):E11.

41. Wakao N, Imagama S, Ito Z, et al. Clinical outcome of treatments for spinal dural arteriovenous fistulas: results of multivariate analysis and review of the literature. Spine (Phila Pa 1976) 2012;37(6):482–8.

42. Ruiz-Juretschke F, Perez-Calvo JM, Castro E, et al. A single-center, long-term study of spinal dural arteriovenous fistulas with multidisciplinary treatment. J Clin Neurosci 2011;18(12):1662–6.

43. Goyal A, Cesare J, Lu VM, et al. Outcomes following surgical versus endovascular treatment of spinal dural arteriovenous fistula: a systematic review and meta-analysis. J Neurol Neurosurg Psychiatry 2019;90(10):1139–46.

44. Li J, Zeng G, Zhi X, et al. Pediatric perimedullary arteriovenous fistula: clinical features and endovascular treatments. J Neurointerv Surg 2019;11(4):411–5.

45. Cho WS, Wang KC, Phi JH, et al. Pediatric spinal arteriovenous malformations and fistulas: a single institute's experience. Childs Nerv Syst 2016;32(5):811–8.

46. Phadke RV, Bhattacharyya A, Handique A, et al. Endovascular treatment in spinal perimedullary arteriovenous fistula. Interv Neuroradiol 2014;20(3):357–67.

47. Lv X, Li Y, Yang X, et al. Endovascular embolization for symptomatic perimedullary AVF and intramedullary AVM: a series and a literature review. Neuroradiology 2012;54(4):349–59.

48. Casasco A, Guimaraens L, Cuellar H, et al. Direct percutaneous venous puncture and embolization of giant perimedullary arteriovenous fistulas. AJNR Am J Neuroradiol 2011;32(1):E10–3.

49. Meng X, Zhang H, Wang Y, et al. Perimedullary arteriovenous fistulas in pediatric patients: clinical, angiographical, and therapeutic experiences in a series of 19 cases. Childs Nerv Syst 2010;26(7):889–96.

50. Cho KT, Lee DY, Chung CK, et al. Treatment of spinal cord perimedullary arteriovenous fistula: embolization versus surgery. Neurosurgery 2005;56(2):232–41 [discussion 232–41].

51. Oran I, Parildar M, Derbent A. Treatment of slow-flow (type I) perimedullary spinal arteriovenous fistulas with special reference to embolization. AJNR Am J Neuroradiol 2005;26(10):2582–6.

52. Rodesch G, Hurth M, Alvarez H, et al. Spinal cord intradural arteriovenous fistulae: anatomic, clinical, and therapeutic considerations in a series of 32 consecutive patients seen between 1981 and 2000 with emphasis on endovascular therapy. Neurosurgery 2005;57(5):973–83 [discussion 973–83].

53. Gross BA, Du R. Spinal pial (type IV) arteriovenous fistulae: a systematic pooled analysis of demographics, hemorrhage risk, and treatment results. Neurosurgery 2013;73(1):141–51 [discussion 151].

54. Kalani MY, Ahmed AS, Martirosyan NL, et al. Surgical and endovascular treatment of pediatric spinal arteriovenous malformations. World Neurosurg 2012;78(3–4):348–54.

55. Alomari AI, Chaudry G, Rodesch G, et al. Complex spinal-paraspinal fast-flow lesions in CLOVES syndrome: analysis of clinical and imaging findings in 6 patients. AJNR Am J Neuroradiol 2011;32(10):1812–7.

56. Corkill RA, Mitsos AP, Molyneux AJ. Embolization of spinal intramedullary arteriovenous malformations using the liquid embolic agent, Onyx: a single-center experience in a series of 17 patients. J Neurosurg Spine 2007;7(5):478–85.

57. Cullen S, Alvarez H, Rodesch G, et al. Spinal arteriovenous shunts presenting before 2 years of age: analysis of 13 cases. Childs Nerv Syst 2006;22(9):1103–10.

58. Gross BA, Du R. Spinal glomus (type II) arteriovenous malformations: a pooled analysis of hemorrhage risk and results of intervention. Neurosurgery 2013;72(1):25–32 [discussion 32].

59. Wilson DA, Abla AA, Uschold TD, et al. Multimodality treatment of conus medullaris arteriovenous malformations: 2 decades of experience with combined endovascular and microsurgical treatments. Neurosurgery 2012;71(1):100–8.

60. Loh Y, Duckwiler GR, Onyx Trial I. A prospective, multicenter, randomized trial of the Onyx liquid embolic system and N-butyl cyanoacrylate embolization of cerebral arteriovenous malformations. Clinical article. J Neurosurg 2010;113(4):733–41.

61. Blackburn SL, Kadkhodayan Y, Ray WZ, et al. Onyx is associated with poor venous penetration in the treatment of spinal dural arteriovenous fistulas. J Neurointerv Surg 2014;6(7):536–40.

Treatment of Pseudotumor Cerebri (Sinus Stenosis)

Shail Thanki, MD, Waldo Guerrero, MD, Maxim Mokin, MD, PhD*

KEYWORDS

• Gradient • Pseudotumor cerebri • Stenting • Sinus

KEY POINTS

• Idiopathic intracranial hypertension is a diagnosis that requires vigilant attention and multidisciplinary approach.
• The current literature recommends acetazolamide as the first-line treatment for those patients who are able to take this medication.
• Venous stenosis stenting is an emerging treatment option that has shown good outcomes for symptomatic improvement in headache, vision loss, and tinnitus.

INTRODUCTION

Idiopathic intracranial hypertension (IIH), pseudotumor cerebri (PTC), and benign intracranial hypertension are all terms used to describe a neurologic syndrome characterized by elevated intracranial pressure (ICP), headache, vision loss, and absence of underlying mass lesion and infection.[1] The first cases of IIH were described by Heinrich Quincke in 1893 in a paper describing patients with increased ICP due to increase in cerebrospinal fluid (CSF) secretion mediated by autonomic nervous system. Max Nonne was the first to coin the term "pseudotumor cerebri."[2] Foley later introduced the term "benign intracranial hypertension." Since the 1980s, the approach to this condition has largely changed requiring aggressive management to avoid permanent sequelae mostly due to visual disturbances. Hence, the term "benign" has largely been replaced by the current moniker of IIH.[2] More recently, a revised diagnostic criterion was proposed for PTC to incorporate advances in neuroimaging and patients with secondary causes. This classification described IIH as primary PTC, whereas those with identifiable causes, such as venous sinus thrombosis, medications, and medical conditions, are secondary.[3]

EPIDEMIOLOGY

In the general population, the incidence of IIH is 1 to 2 per 100,000. IIH is 10 times more common in women than in men, and obesity increases the risk of developing IIH approximately 20-fold. The incidences increase to 12 to 32 per 100,000 in obese women of childbearing age.[4,5] In pediatric population, the incidence rate is similar in both sexes in the prepubertal age. However, the incidence in obese adolescent females is almost twice that of obese adolescent males. Obesity was a common major risk for both sexes because more than 80% of IIH cases in those aged 12 to 15 years were in obese patients.[6]

PATHOPHYSIOLOGY

Although, the first cases of IIH were described more than 100 years ago, the pathogenesis remains still unclear. Multiple theories have been proposed describing different mechanisms such as parenchymal edema, increased cerebral blood volume, excessive CSF production, venous outflow obstruction, and compromised CSF absorption.[7–10] In addition, it has been postulated that obesity plays a role, given its prevalence in this population of patients.

Department of Neurosurgery and Brain Repair, University of South Florida, Tampa, FL, USA
* Corresponding author. University of South Florida Neurosurgery, 2 Tampa General Circle, 7th floor, Tampa, FL 33606.
E-mail address: mokin@usf.edu

Neurosurg Clin N Am 33 (2022) 207–214
https://doi.org/10.1016/j.nec.2021.11.002
1042-3680/22/© 2021 Elsevier Inc. All rights reserved.

Increased Cerebrospinal Fluid Production

It has been proposed that increased CSF production has a role to play in PTC; however, in patients with CSF hypersecretion with known causes such as choroid plexus hyperplasia, patients often develop ventriculomegaly and hydrocephalus. However, the normal or decreased ventricular size found in patients with IIH suggests that there is no increased CSF production in most of the patients.[4]

Decreased Cerebrospinal Fluid Reabsorption

Some studies have demonstrated an abnormally increased outflow resistance indicating a potential defect through the arachnoid granulations into the cortical venous sinuses. Cerebral venous stenosis, particularly in the bilateral or dominant transverse sinuses, is an imaging finding seen in most, if not all, patients with IIH.[11] According to one theory, there is a positive feedback loop between increased ICP from an unclear inciting event causing extramural compression of the venous sinuses and intracranial venous congestion caused by outflow obstruction.[12]

It is proposed that obesity elevates intra-abdominal pressure, which causes increase in pleural and cardiac filling pressures. This is in turn leads to decreased venous return from the brain, subsequently causing less CSF absorption.[13] Studies have also suggested a link between obesity and inflammatory markers such as cytokines, interleukins, and leptin.[14,15]

CLINICAL FEATURES

A typical presentation of IIH is that of an overweight female of childbearing age who complains of headache and is typically found to have papilledema on funduscopic examination. However, the clinical presentation sometimes varies among patients. In one retrospective study, 72% patients with IIH had presented with visual disturbances but only 44% patients had papilledema on examination.[16] In the Idiopathic Intracranial Hypertension Treatment Trial (IIHTT), 84% to 92% of patients reported headache.[17] Headaches can vary in character and severity and can sometimes mimic other primary headache disorders such as migraine or tension type. Features like retrobulbar pain and mild pain with eye movement or globe compression are somewhat more specific for IIH. In some patients, the pain follows a trigeminal or cervical nerve root distribution, although neck stiffness and back pain are also commonly reported.[18] Among children, headache is a less common feature with about 29% of children with IIH not reporting headache according to one study.[19] Visual disturbances are the

hallmark of IIH, and presence of vision loss in the setting of headache should highly raise the suspicion of IIH. For many patients, it may be the presenting symptom. Most commonly reported visual symptoms are transient visual obscurations (68%–72%) lasting seconds at a time and can be unilateral or bilateral. Less commonly, some patients will have a fulminant course with rapid development of vision loss within 4 weeks of onset of symptoms.[20] Rarely, patients present with diplopia due to unilateral or bilateral cranial nerve VI palsy (18%–38%).[17,21] Other less common symptoms include tinnitus, back pain, neck pain, and photopsia.[17]

DIAGNOSIS

Classically, IIH is diagnosed as a triad of headache, visual changes, and papilledema. However, over the recent years, due to development of imaging and diagnostic tools along with better understanding of the disease, IIH is now diagnosed according to modified Dandy criteria (**Box 1**).[22] The IIHT algorithm of 2014 uses the same requirements except that the threshold for the increased CSF opening pressure is lowered to greater than 200 mm H_2O (**Box 2**).[17] In patients suspected to have PTC, MRI of the brain and lumbar puncture with measurement of opening pressure are usually performed to rule out secondary causes. A thorough evaluation of the medication history, genetic and endocrine disorders, and other medical disorders should be performed before giving a patient the diagnosis of primary PTC.

MANAGEMENT
Medical Therapy

The first line treatment of IIH is medical management and weight loss. In a randomized trial (IIHTT) of 165 patients with IIH and mild vision loss,

---

Box 1

Modified Dandy criteria for the diagnosis of pseudotumor cerebri[22]

Dandy Criteria for the Diagnosis of Pseudotumor Cerebri

- Signs and symptoms of increased intracranial pressure (headache, nausea, vomiting, transient visual obscurations, papilledema)
- No localizing neurologic signs except for unilateral or bilateral cranial nerve VI palsy
- Elevated CSF opening pressure without cytologic or chemical abnormalities
- Normal to small ventricles as evidenced by computed tomography/MRI

Box 2
Idiopathic Intracranial Hypertension Treatment Trial modified Dandy criteria[23]

- Signs and symptoms of increased intracranial pressure
- Absence of localizing findings on neurologic examination
- Absence of deformity, displacement, or obstruction of the ventricular system and otherwise normal neurodiagnostic studies, except for evidence of increased cerebrospinal fluid pressure (>200 mm H_2O). Abnormal neuroimaging except for empty sella turcica, optic nerve sheath with filled out CSF spaces, and smooth-walled non-flow-related venous sinus stenosis or collapse should lead to another diagnosis
- Awake and alert
- No other cause of increased ICP

  If the CSF opening pressure was 200–250 mm H_2O, at least one of the following is required:

  - Pulse synchronous tinnitus
  - Cranial nerve VI palsy
  - Frisen grade II papilledema
  - Echography of drusen negative and no other disc anomalies mimicking disc edema present
  - Magnetic resonance venography with lateral sinus collapse/stenosis preferably using autotriggered elliptical centric ordered technique
  - Partially empty sella on coronal or sagittal views and optic nerve sheaths with filled out CSF spaces next to the globe on T2-weighted axial scans

treatment with carbonic anhydrase inhibitor (acetazolamide) showed modest improvement in a perimetric measurement of global visual field loss, along with improvements in papilledema grade, CSF pressure, and vision-related quality of life at 6 months.[24] Topiramate is another medication that has shown benefit in patients with IIH because of its mild carbonic anhydrase activity and effectiveness in preventing migraine headaches. In addition, it also carries the side effect profile of causing weight loss, which may be beneficial to these patients.[25] Alternatively, loop diuretics such as furosemide and chlorthalidone have been used as stand-alone treatment for those unable to tolerate topiramate or acetazolamide or in combination with these medications.[26] In those

patients who continue to remain symptomatic despite maximum medical therapy or those patients who do not tolerate acetazolamide, several surgical options exist including CSF diversion, optic nerve sheath fenestration (ONSF), bariatric surgery, and venous sinus stenting (VSS).[27] However, randomized controlled trials need to be performed for these surgical options to determine the best practices in medically refractory IIH.

Surgical Treatment

Surgical treatment is often reserved for those patients who fail maximum medical therapy or are intolerant to or are noncompliant with medical therapy and are at risk of developing vision loss as evidenced by worsening vision field defect or presence of visual acuity loss attributed to papilledema.[28] Two main procedures in IIH treatment are optic nerve sheath fenestration and CSF flow diversion procedures. Cerebral venous stenting is an alternative treatment of IIH that has shown promising results in recent studies.[29,30]

Optic Nerve Sheath Fenestration

ONSF is an effective treatment in patients who have progressive vision loss despite medical therapy. The procedure involves creating slits in the edematous optic nerve sheath and allowing CSF egress into the orbit. ONSF has shown postoperative improvement in patients' visual fields and visual acuity.[31] In a large case series, visual acuity stabilized or improved in 94% of patients who underwent ONSF, whereas visual field stabilized or improved in 88% of patients.[32] The primary goal of ONSF in IIH is to preserve vision, but its impact on the ICP improvement remains minimal.

Cerebrospinal Fluid Flow Diversion

Serial lumbar punctures have been performed in patients to rapidly relieve intracranial hypertension and decrease ICP primarily because of the proposed mechanism of increased CSF production in IIH. However, these are not useful long-term treatment options in patients with IIH and are useful temporizing measures as a prelude to surgery.[33] The most common definitive surgical treatment of IIH is placement of ventriculoperitoneal shunt or lumboperitoneal shunt. A large meta-analysis consisting of 17 studies including 435 patients who underwent CSF flow diversion for treatment of IIH showed good success in relieving symptoms of headache and signs of papilledema. The investigators reported that 86% patients experienced improvement in their headaches, whereas 70% patients had improvement in their papilledema. Changes in visual acuity showed less improvement than other symptoms.[34] Complications were reported in 7.6% patients and included shunt infection, subdural hematoma, tonsillar herniation, and CSF fistula.[34]

Venous Sinus Stenting

Dural venous sinus stenosis is a common finding in patients with IIH. One study reported incidences of transverse sinus stenosis in IIH to range from 10% to 90% compared with 6.8% in general population.[35] Another study reported 93% of patients with IIH to have bilateral venous sinus stenosis compared with 7% on magnetic resonance venography (MRV).[36] Transverse sinus stenting is a relatively new approach that has been used to treat IIH when sinus stenosis is seen on imaging. However, the relationship between IIH and transverse sinus stenosis has been controversial largely because it is unclear if venous stenosis is a cause of IIH or occurs as a result of this. Higgins and colleagues[37] were the first to describe VSS for refractory IIH. The investigators reported a patient with IIH with partial bilateral transverse sinus stenosis with a pressure gradient across the stenotic segments. After placement of a stent across one of the stenotic segments, significant reduction was noted in the pressure gradient with improvement in headaches and resolution of papilledema.[37] Buell and colleagues[38] published evidence of venous stenosis as a manifestation of IIH. The investigators reported a case of a patient with IIH who had improvement in the transstenosis pressure gradient and venous stenosis after a high-volume lumbar puncture (HVLP). Recurrence of venous stenosis coincided with the opening pressure on HVLP. Venous sinus stent placement resulted in clinical improvement. The investigators hypothesized that endovascular stenting may obliterate a positive feedback loop involving transstenosis pressure gradient.[38]

The preoperative workup for VSS includes ophthalmologic evaluation, lumbar puncture, and MRV (**Figs. 1** and **2**). During the cerebral venogram, pressures are obtained at superior sagittal sinus (SSS), torcula, bilateral transverse sinus, sigmoid sinus, and cervical internal jugular vein. Most investigators reported stenting in patients with pressure gradient 8 cm H_2O or greater. In one of the ongoing clinical trial, patients with IIH with CSF opening pressure greater than 25 cm H_2O, pressure gradient greater than 8, and venographic evidence

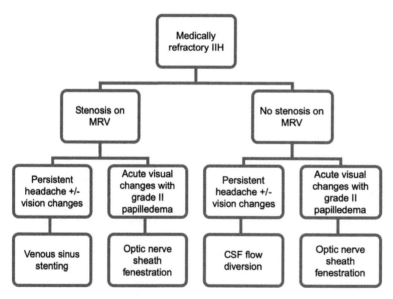

Fig. 1. Flowchart algorithm for treatment and management of medically refractory IIH. MRV is an excellent utility to assess for venous sinus stenosis. MRV should be performed as part of the initial workup for the IIH. For those patients who have evidence of venous sinus stenosis on MRV, persistent headaches, and elevated opening pressures objectively measured by lumbar puncture, with or without visual changes, VSS should be considered for treatment. Long-term follow-up is recommended if patient experiences resolution of headache and stable vision. However, if patient's vision continues to deteriorate, then CSF diversion should be considered as the next therapeutic option. For those patients who have no evidence of venous sinus stenosis on MRV and persistent headaches and high opening pressure, with or without vision changes, CSF flow diversion is recommended as the most appropriate surgical option. ONSF is recommended in patients with acute visual changes and grade II papilledema. If patient's visual complaints remain stable, continued long-term follow-up is recommended. If visual complaints persist after ONSF for patients with evidence of venous sinus stenosis on MRV, practitioners should consider a trial of VSS. If VSS is selected as the therapeutic option and fails to control visual changes, CSF flow diversion can alternatively be offered to the patient for symptomatic relief. For those patients with acute visual changes whose symptoms are not relieved by ONSF and who have no evidence of venous sinus stenosis on MRV, CSF flow diversion is recommended.[48] However, a retrospective study has shown benefit of VSS in patients with IIH with acute vision loss leading to possibility of stenting as a first-line treatment option.[43]

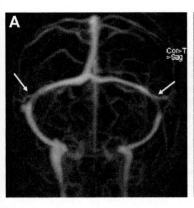
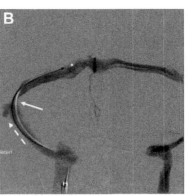

Fig. 2. Magnetic resonance venogram of head showing stenosis of the right transverse-sigmoid sinus. (*A*). Magnetic resonance venogram, coronal view, showing bilateral stenosis of the transverse-sigmoid junction (*arrows*) in a patient with suspected IIH. (*B*) Digital subtraction angiogram, venous injection. The white arrow points to stenosis of the right transverse-sigmoid junction. Adjacent to it is a venous diverticulum (*dashed arrow*). A microcatheter can be seen within the right transverse sinus to measure venous gradient.

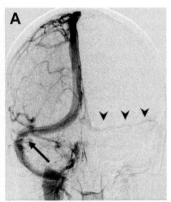
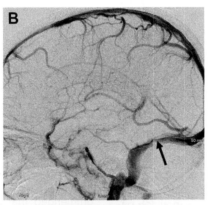
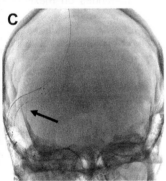
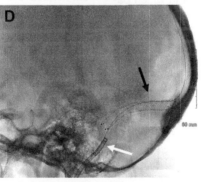
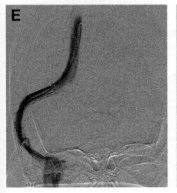
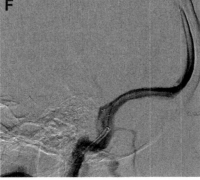

Fig. 3. Stenting of venous sinus stenosis. Diagnostic cerebral angiogram, (A) anteroposterior and (B) lateral projections, showing stenosis of dominant right transverse sigmoid sinus junction (*arrows*). The left transverse sinus is hypoplastic in this case (*arrowheads*). Fluoroscopy, (*C*) anteroposterior and (*D*) lateral projections, showing deployed stent (*arrows*) to treat the underlying stenosis. Venogram, (*E*) anteroposterior and (*F*) lateral projections, confirming successful angiographic result postintervention.

of sinus stenosis greater than 50% were included (Venous Sinus Stenting With the River Stent in IIH trial). In most studies, unilateral VSS was done despite the presence of bilateral stenosis, with the dominant side or the side with greater degree of stenosis being the preferred choice.[39] A meta-analysis of 143 patients with IIH done by Puffer and colleagues reported 93% receiving a unilateral stent and 69% of the stents were placed in the right transverse-sigmoid sinus (**Fig. 3**).[30] Antiplatelet therapy was used in the periprocedural and postprocedural periods with aspirin and clopidogrel usually started 4 to 5 days before the procedure and continued for a period of 3 to 6 months; this was followed by aspirin therapy.[40] Duration of aspirin therapy has ranged from 3 months to lifelong use in various studies.

Several studies have analyzed the efficacy and the safety profile of VSS in IIH. In a review of 185 patients by Starke and colleagues,[41] 78.3% of patients reported resolution or improvement in headaches; 86.5% of patients who had presented with visual changes had reported improvement or restoration of their normal vision after the procedure, whereas papilledema resolved in all but 5 patients (94.4%). Improvement in tinnitus was noted in 92.9% patients, whereas the mean transstenotic pressure gradient improved from 20.1 mm Hg to 4.4 mm Hg following the VSS.[41] A case series by Matloob and colleagues[42] demonstrated immediate reduction in ICP with VSS that was sustained at 24 hours. This was the first study in which patients had real-time intraparenchymal pressure monitoring during VSS.[42] In another study, VSS was performed in patients with IIH with acute vision loss and resulted in satisfactory clinical outcome with improvement in vision in 80% patients.[43]

A 2015 meta-analysis of VSS by Satti and colleagues[34] reported a 7.4% complication rate, with 2.9% having a major complication of subdural hematoma requiring surgical decompression. Another possible complication is cerebellar hemorrhage, and its risk is inversely associated with the age of the patient.[44] With any vascular stenting, the most feared complication is acute thrombosis and stenosis of stent. However, none of the studies have reported complete occlusion, but studies have reported stent-adjacent stenosis (SAS), which is due to stenosis in the sinus adjacent to the stent, rather than the in-stent stenosis, which is seen in arterial stents. It has been observed that incidence of SAS is higher with larger stent diameters.[45] SAS commonly manifests weeks after VSS and involves susceptible regions of the sinus and is typically seen rostral to the stent but not caudal to the stent.[12] Even though the reported incidence is 18% in VSS, only ~10% are symptomatic, which require further treatment or intervention.[46] Overall, the rate of other complications is 5.4%, which includes femoral pseudoaneurysm, subdural hematoma, transient hearing loss, and stent migration.[41]

Several other studies have shown lower complication rates with VSS than with shunting, but the clinical outcomes are not easily comparable.[47]

SUMMARY

IIH remains a diagnosis that requires vigilant attention and multidisciplinary approach especially in high-risk patient populations of obese, childbearing age women and those with symptoms of visual changes and headache because the risks of permanent vision loss and significant disability are high. Improvement in imaging along with new diagnostic criteria has helped to better categorize patients and individualize treatment. The current literature recommends acetazolamide as the first-line treatment for those patients who are able to take this medication. Second-line agents such as topiramate and loop diuretics are available for those who are unable to tolerate acetazolamide.

In patients with refractory IIH and specifically with vision loss, surgical options of ONSF and CSF flow diversion with shunts remain the viable options. VSS is an emerging treatment option that has shown good outcomes for symptomatic improvement in headache, vision loss, and tinnitus. It is recommended that patient continues on maximum medical therapy under the care of a headache specialist with expertise in IIH because incidence of other primary headaches in these patients is commonly seen. Although the evidence of VSS in IIH is promising, further studies are required to compare its efficacy with ONSF and CSF flow diversion, which will help in further selecting the best candidates for stent placement and hence creating specific best-practice guidelines for the treatment of the medically refractory IIH. There are 2 ongoing clinical trials (RIVER study and Operative Procedures vs. Endovascular Neurosurgery for Untreated Pseudotumor Trial [OPEN-UP] trial) that will determine the role of VSS in treating patients with IIH and provide the best evidence to determine the optimal treatment option.

CLINICS CARE POINTS

- Visual disturbances are present in 72% of patients with IIH while only 44% have papilledema. Meanwhile, headache is reported in 84-92% of patients with IIH.

- Surgical therapy is typically reserved for patients who fail medical therapy or those who are at risk of developing vision loss.
- Venous sinus stenting is an emerging treatment generally preferred in patients with persistent headaches +/- vision changes.
- 78% patients reported improvement in headache after VSS while 86% patients noted improvement in visual disturbances.
- Complication of VSS includes subdural and intraparenchymal hemorrhage, stenosis or occlusion of the stent and requires anti-platelet therapy for a short duration.

DISCLOSURE

M. Mokin—Grants: Principal investigator NIH R21NS109575; Consultant: Medtronic, Cerenovus; Stock options: Brain Q, Endostream, Serenity medical, Synchron. S.T. and W. Guerrero: none.

REFERENCES

1. Burkett JG, Ailani J. An Up to Date Review of Pseudotumor Cerebri Syndrome. Curr Neurol Neurosci Rep 2018;18(6):33.
2. Johnston I. The historical development of the pseudotumor concept. Neurosurg Focus 2001;11(2):E2.
3. Friedman DI, Liu GT, Digre KB. Revised diagnostic criteria for the pseudotumor cerebri syndrome in adults and children. Neurology 2013;81(13): 1159–65.
4. Baykan B, Ekizoglu E, Altiokka Uzun G. An update on the pathophysiology of idiopathic intracranial hypertension alias pseudotumor cerebri. Agri 2015; 27(2):63–72.
5. Kesler A, Stolovic N, Bluednikov Y, et al. The incidence of idiopathic intracranial hypertension in Israel from 2005 to 2007: results of a nationwide survey. Eur J Neurol 2014;21(8):1055–9.
6. Matthews YY, Dean F, Lim MJ, et al. Pseudotumor cerebri syndrome in childhood: incidence, clinical profile and risk factors in a national prospective population-based cohort study. Arch Dis Child 2017;102(8):715–21.
7. Iencean SM. Simultaneous hypersecretion of CSF and of brain interstitial fluid causes idiopathic intracranial hypertension. Med Hypotheses 2003;61(5–6):529–32.
8. Johnston I. Reduced C.S.F. absorption syndrome. Reappraisal of benign intracranial hypertension and related conditions. Lancet 1973;2(7826):418–21.
9. Malm J, Kristensen B, Markgren P, et al. CSF hydrodynamics in idiopathic intracranial hypertension: a long-term study. Neurology 1992;42(4):851–8.
10. Markey KA, Mollan SP, Jensen RH, et al. Understanding idiopathic intracranial hypertension: mechanisms, management, and future directions. Lancet Neurol 2016;15(1):78–91.
11. Riggeal BD, Bruce BB, Saindane AM, et al. Clinical course of idiopathic intracranial hypertension with transverse sinus stenosis. Neurology 2013;80(3): 289–95.
12. Fargen KM. A unifying theory explaining venous sinus stenosis and recurrent stenosis following venous sinus stenting in patients with idiopathic intracranial hypertension. J Neurointerv Surg 2021; 13(7):587–92.
13. Subramaniam S, Fletcher WA. Obesity and Weight Loss in Idiopathic Intracranial Hypertension: A Narrative Review. J Neuroophthalmol 2017;37(2): 197–205.
14. Edwards LJ, Sharrack B, Ismail A, et al. Increased levels of interleukins 2 and 17 in the cerebrospinal fluid of patients with idiopathic intracranial hypertension. Am J Clin Exp Immunol 2013;2(3):234–44.
15. Lampl Y, Eshel Y, Kessler A, et al. Serum leptin level in women with idiopathic intracranial hypertension. J Neurol Neurosurg Psychiatr 2002;72(5):642–3.
16. Cappuzzo JM, Hess RM, Morrison JF, et al. Transverse venous stenting for the treatment of idiopathic intracranial hypertension, or pseudotumor cerebri. Neurosurg Focus 2018;45(1):E11.
17. Wall M, Kupersmith MJ, Kieburtz KD, et al. The idiopathic intracranial hypertension treatment trial: clinical profile at baseline. JAMA Neurol 2014;71(6): 693–701.
18. Wall M. The headache profile of idiopathic intracranial hypertension. Cephalalgia 1990;10(6):331–5.
19. Lim M, Kurian M, Penn A, et al. Visual failure without headache in idiopathic intracranial hypertension. Arch Dis Child 2005;90(2):206–10.
20. Thambisetty M, Lavin PJ, Newman NJ, et al. Fulminant idiopathic intracranial hypertension. Neurology 2007;68(3):229–32.
21. Chari C, Rao NS. Benign intracranial hypertension–its unusual manifestations. Headache 1991;31(9): 599–600.
22. Smith JL. Whence pseudotumor cerebri? J Clin Neuroophthalmol 1985;5(1):55–6.
23. Wall M, Friedman DI, Corbett JJ, et al. Revised diagnostic criteria for the pseudotumor cerebri syndrome in adults and children. Neurology 2014;83(2):198–200.
24. Wall M, McDermott MP, Kieburtz KD, et al. Effect of acetazolamide on visual function in patients with idiopathic intracranial hypertension and mild visual loss: the idiopathic intracranial hypertension treatment trial. Jama 2014;311(16):1641–51.
25. Celebisoy N, Gökçay F, Sirin H, et al. Treatment of idiopathic intracranial hypertension: topiramate vs acetazolamide, an open-label study. Acta Neurol Scand 2007;116(5):322–7.

26. Matthews YY. Drugs used in childhood idiopathic or benign intracranial hypertension. Arch Dis Child Educ Pract Ed 2008;93(1):19–25.

27. Mukherjee N, Bhatti MT. Update on the surgical management of idiopathic intracranial hypertension. Curr Neurol Neurosci Rep 2014;14(3):438.

28. Corbett JJ, Thompson HS. The rational management of idiopathic intracranial hypertension. Arch Neurol 1989;46(10):1049–51.

29. Ahmed RM, Wilkinson M, Parker GD, et al. Transverse sinus stenting for idiopathic intracranial hypertension: a review of 52 patients and of model predictions. AJNR Am J Neuroradiol 2011;32(8): 1408–14.

30. Puffer RC, Mustafa W, Lanzino G. Venous sinus stenting for idiopathic intracranial hypertension: a review of the literature. J Neurointerv Surg 2013; 5(5):483–6.

31. Feldon SE. Visual outcomes comparing surgical techniques for management of severe idiopathic intracranial hypertension. Neurosurg Focus 2007; 23(5):E6.

32. Banta JT, Farris BK. Pseudotumor cerebri and optic nerve sheath decompression. Ophthalmology 2000; 107(10):1907–12.

33. Huna-Baron R, Kupersmith MJ. Idiopathic intracranial hypertension in pregnancy. J Neurol 2002; 249(8):1078–81.

34. Satti SR, Leishangthem L, Chaudry MI. Meta-Analysis of CSF Diversion Procedures and Dural Venous Sinus Stenting in the Setting of Medically Refractory Idiopathic Intracranial Hypertension. AJNR Am J Neuroradiol 2015;36(10):1899–904.

35. Elder BD, Goodwin CR, Kosztowski TA, et al. Venous sinus stenting is a valuable treatment for fulminant idiopathic intracranial hypertension. J Clin Neurosci 2015;22(4):685–9.

36. Farb RI, Vanek I, Scott JN, et al. Idiopathic intracranial hypertension: the prevalence and morphology of sinovenous stenosis. Neurology 2003;60(9):1418–24.

37. Higgins JN, Owler BK, Cousins C, et al. Venous sinus stenting for refractory benign intracranial hypertension. Lancet 2002;359(9302):228–30.

38. Buell TJ, Raper DMS, Pomeraniec IJ, et al. Transient resolution of venous sinus stenosis after high-volume lumbar puncture in a patient with idiopathic intracranial hypertension. J Neurosurg 2018;129(1): 153–6.

39. Kanagalingam S, Subramanian PS. Cerebral venous sinus stenting for pseudotumor cerebri: A review. Saudi J Ophthalmol 2015;29(1):3–8.

40. Liu KC, Starke RM, Durst CR, et al. Venous sinus stenting for reduction of intracranial pressure in IIH: a prospective pilot study. J Neurosurg 2017; 127(5):1126–33.

41. Starke RM, Wang T, Ding D, et al. Endovascular Treatment of Venous Sinus Stenosis in Idiopathic Intracranial Hypertension: Complications, Neurological Outcomes, and Radiographic Results. ScientificWorldJournal 2015;2015:140408.

42. Matloob SA, Toma AK, Thompson SD, et al. Effect of venous stenting on intracranial pressure in idiopathic intracranial hypertension. Acta Neurochir (Wien) 2017;159(8):1429–37.

43. Zehri AH, Lee KE, Kartchner J, et al. Efficacy of dural venous sinus stenting in treating idiopathic intracranial hypertension with acute vision loss. Neuroradiol J 2021. 19714009211026923.

44. Lavoie P, Audet M, Gariepy JL, et al. Severe cerebellar hemorrhage following transverse sinus stenting for idiopathic intracranial hypertension. Interv Neuroradiol 2018;24(1):100–5.

45. El Mekabaty A, Pearl MS, Moghekar A, et al. Midterm assessment of transverse sinus stent patency in 104 patients treated for intracranial hypertension secondary to dural sinus stenosis. J NeuroInterventional Surg 2021;13(2):182–6.

46. Raper D, Buell TJ, Ding D, et al. Pattern of pressure gradient alterations after venous sinus stenting for idiopathic intracranial hypertension predicts stent-adjacent stenosis: a proposed classification system. J Neurointerv Surg 2018;10(4):391–5.

47. Arac A, Lee M, Steinberg GK, et al. Efficacy of endovascular stenting in dural venous sinus stenosis for the treatment of idiopathic intracranial hypertension. Neurosurg Focus 2009;27(5):E14.

48. Giridharan N, Patel SK, Ojugbeli A, et al. Understanding the complex pathophysiology of idiopathic intracranial hypertension and the evolving role of venous sinus stenting: a comprehensive review of the literature. Neurosurg Focus 2018;45(1):E10.

Novel Innovation in Flow Diversion
Surface Modifications

Joseph S. Hudson, MD, Michael J. Lang, MD, Bradley A. Gross, MD*

KEYWORDS

- Stent • Intracranial aneurysm • Sub-arachnoid hemorrhage • Flow diversion

KEY POINTS

- The initial short and medium-term outcomes data suggest similar rates of angiographic aneurysm occlusion with antithrombotic surface-modified devices.
- Although heterogenous, preliminary data suggest a lower rate of stent-associated ischemic events in patients treated with surface-modified flow diverting devices.
- Several cases of mono antiplatelet therapy in the setting of aneurysm treatment with surface-modified or coated flow diverters have been described with varying success.
- Surface modification of flow diverters with antithrombotic enzymatically active glycoproteins has shown in vitro and in vivo antithrombogenic properties.

INTRODUCTION

Flow diversion is a frequently used endovascular modality for the treatment of certain intracranial aneurysms. The cylindrical porous metal mesh wires divert blood flow from the aneurysm sac and ultimately provide a scaffold for endothelial growth.[1] The stent structure typically provides around 30% to 35% metal coverage. Aneurysm occlusion then occurs in the order of weeks to months. Initial trials performed in 2011 demonstrated high rates of complete angiographic obliteration in difficult to treat and wide-necked aneurysms.[2] Several flow diverting devices initially became available, including the Pipeline Embolization Device (PED, ev3/Covidien, Irvine, California, approved in 2011), the Silk flow diverter (SILK; Bal Extrusion, Montmorency, France, approved in the EU in 2008), and the Surpass flow diverter (Stryker Neurovascular, Freemont, California, approved in the EU.) The technology has now become the standard of care for a variety of aneurysm morphologies and locations. Off-label use of flow diverters, is commonplace in many institutions, and has been extended to ruptured aneurysms. However, there remains a risk of aneurysmal rebleeding given the speed aneurysm occlusion and requisite dual antiplatelet therapy after deployment. In fact, patients with ruptured aneurysms treated with flow diversion had a reported higher rate of aneurysmal rebleed (4%–5%) when compared with the 2.7% rate of rebleeding after endovascular coiling reported in the ISAT trial.[3–5] Moreover, there remains a risk of hemorrhagic complications during subsequent neurosurgical procedures associated with aneurysm rupture. In a single institution study of 443 patients with ruptured intracranial aneurysms, those who required dual antiplatelet therapy were more likely to have radiographic hemorrhage after placement of external ventricular drains (odds ratio (OR): 4.92, $P = .0001$).[6] This finding was extended to patients receiving ventriculoperitoneal shunts after posthemorrhagic hydrocephalus in that same cohort (OR: 31.23, $P = .0001$).[7] Given these risks, there has been a concerted effort from practicing neurosurgeons, device companies, and biomedical engineers to develop

Department of Neurosurgery, University of Pittsburgh Medical Center, 200 Lothrop Street, Pittsburgh, PA, USA
* Corresponding author.
E-mail address: grossb2@upmc.edu
Twitter: @js_hudson (J.S.H.)

Neurosurg Clin N Am 33 (2022) 215–218
https://doi.org/10.1016/j.nec.2021.11.004

devices which are inherently antithrombotic. The remainder of this article will focus on describing these devices and discussing the *in vivo* and *in vitro* data regarding their efficacy.

DEVICES AND SURFACE MODIFICATIONS
Pipeline Embolization Flex Device with Shield Technology

The PED Flex with "SHIELD" technology, a so-called third-generation flow diverter, was developed and subsequently introduced in 2014. The key design feature distinguishing it from its "bare metal" predecessors is a phosphorylcholine polymer covalently bonded to the metal pipeline braid (75% Cobalt Chrome, 25% Platinum/Tungsten). In vitro scanning electron microscopy of the device surface when placed in human blood artificial flow models has revealed reduced microthrombus formation.[8] Mechanistically, this coating affords the device biomimetic properties, specifically simulating the cell phospholipid membrane. The recently published single-arm multicenter observational study (SHIELD), sought to ascertain the rates of angiographic aneurysm occlusion and major stroke in the affected territory in aneurysm treated with the device. In 151 patients treated at seven centers, 85% of patients developed angiographic occlusion at 12 months. Neurologic complications, including strokes, were limited to 6.6% of patients.[9] It is important to note, that in this series, patients were still maintained on a regimen of dual antiplatelet agents for 6 months. In a separate series of 50 patients treated with the shield device, Galdamez MM et al. reported 6 cases of in-stent thrombosis.[10] In an interesting demonstration of reduced thrombogenicity, Pikis and colleagues obtained MRI's demonstrating a reduced level of silent diffusion restriction within 72 hours after aneurysm treatment with a shield device.[11] We look forward to a more complete understanding of the efficacy of PED with shield technology as additional longer term follow-up data emerges.

Derivo Embolization Device

The Derivo embolization device (DED, Acandis GmbH, Pforzheim, Germany) was introduced in 2016 and consists of 24 Nitinol wires with radiopaque platinum core loops. The device is modified with a 50 nm titanium oxide surface finish (coating) that theoretically reduces friction during delivery and expansion, and ultimately thrombogenicity. Taschner and colleagues report that in a prospective multi-center study of 119 patients the major morbidity rate (modified Rankin scale greater than 3) was 3.1% and the major stroke

rate was 4%.[12] Aneurysm occlusion at 1 year was achieved in 89% of patients. In the Brazilian multicenter BRAIDED trial, there was a reported "major adverse event" rate of 5.5%, and again an 89% rate of angiographic occlusion at 1 year.[13] Long-term outcomes data are forthcoming.

Phenox Flow Modulation Device

The hydrophilic polymer coating technology-enabled p64/p48 flow modulation device (HPC, Phenox GmbH, Bochum, Germany) was introduced in 2017, consists of platinum and nitinol braided wires. It uses a proprietary covalently bonded coating that mimics the vessel wall glycocalyx and inhibits platelet plug formation. In a small clinical series of 28 patients with ruptured and unruptured aneurysms treated with HPC, no patients suffered from clinically significant in-stent thrombosis, though most patients received dual antiplatelet therapy.[14] There were 2 thromboembolic events, but no long term morbidity or mortality. Complete obliteration was reported in 87% of cases, though interestingly, posttreatment DWI-MRI demonstrated hits in 70% of patients. Several series discussed below document the use of mono-antiplatelet therapy with varying results.

Covalently Bonded Thrombomodulin

In 2018, Schumacher and colleagues described the creation of a nanometer-scale coating which served as a platform for the covalent bonding of thrombomodulin, an enzymatically active antithrombotic glycoprotein, to commercially available Pipeline stents.[15] *In vitro* testing revealed reduced rates of thrombin generation, which translates to a less enzymatically active coagulation cascade. *In vivo* placement in animals and scanning electron microscopy postplacement revealed reduced platelet aggregation. The molecular scaffold described in this report may serve as a platform for the covalent bonding of other bioactive antithrombotic molecules.

DISCUSSION

The utilization of flow diverting devices with inherently antithrombotic coatings in humans has started, although there have been few direct comparisons of thrombogenicity between devices. When compared in vitro, the PED with shield technology has demonstrated significantly less thrombogenicity when compared with the P64 device, the Derivo flow diverter, and the bare metal PED.[8] These findings have been similarly described in animal models.[16] In humans, data suggest that the rate of ischemic stroke with PED ranges from approximately 4.7% (IntroPED study) to 6.5% (PUFs trial).[17,18] The reported neurologic complication rate of 6.5% at 1-year follow-up in the SHIELD trial falls within these reported rates of in-stent occlusion in supposedly more thrombogenic stents (older generation devices). However, the first meta-analysis examining the clinical outcomes and rates of angiographic occlusion with flow diverters with surface modifications demonstrated lower rates of serious ischemic events (0.8%–3%) when compared with higher rates associated with the SILK, Surpass, and PED devices with similar rates of angiographic occlusion.[19] Among included studies in the meta-analysis, there were significant differences in antiplatelet regimen, platelet function testing, follow-up imaging, and deployment technique. Additionally, the majority of aneurysms treated were small easy to treat anterior circulation saccular aneurysms. It should be noted that all of the efficacy and safety trials for the devices in question have been performed under the administration of antiplatelet medication.

Despite the lack of data, there have been several reports describing mono-platelet therapy in the setting of aneurysms treated with surface-modified flow diverters. Guzzardi and colleagues describe a 7 patient series of ruptured aneurysms treated with aspirin monotherapy and the Phenox HPC device without documented in-stent thrombosis.[20] On the other hand, in a prospective study of aspirin monotherapy after unruptured aneurysm treatment with the HPC device, ischemic complications occurred in 3 out of 7 patients and the study was halted.[21] The first reported use of aspirin monotherapy in the setting of the PED shield deployment for a ruptured fusiform vertebral artery aneurysm was described by Hanel and colleagues in 2017.[22] They did observe clinically insignificant in-stent thrombosis on posttreatment day 10. Finally, a series from Australia describes the use of the PED with shield technology in the setting of acute subarachnoid hemorrhage without dual antiplatelet therapy. Of the 14 patients treated, 1 suffered a complete in-stent thrombosis, and 1 patient died from an aneurysmal rebleed.[23] These mixed results in these clinical series suggest it is not yet safe to consider mono antiplatelet therapy alone when deploying a modified device.

SUMMARY

Flow diversion is a mainstay of modern endovascular aneurysm treatment. Several molecular surface modifications have been introduced to reduce the thrombogenicity of the stents and avoid dual antiplatelet therapy. Preliminary follow-up data support safety and effectiveness of surface-modified flow diverters. These data also suggest that these devices have lower rates of stent-related ischemia. At present, evidence to support the use of single antiplatelet therapy is not sufficient. The authors of this chapter are hopeful that antithrombotic surface modifications may 1 day allow for less reliance on dual antiplatelet therapy and reduced device-related morbidity.

CLINICS CARE POINTS

- There is limited and mixed data regarding the use of mono antiplatelet therapy and surface-modified flow diverters.
- The evidence to date suggests that surface-modified flow diverters have similar angiographic aneurysm occlusion rates when compared with older generation devices at short to medium-term follow-up intervals.
- There is evidence to suggest that commercially available surface modifications to flow diverters may reduce rates of deployment-related ischemic complications.

DISCLOSURE

B.A. Gross is a consultant for Medtronic and MicroVention.

REFERENCES

1. Starke RM, Turk A, Ding D. Technology developments in endovascular treatment of intracranial aneurysms. J Neurointerv Surg 2016;8(2):135–44.
2. Nelson PK, Lylyk P, Szikora I. The pipeline embolization device for the intracranial treatment of aneurysms trial. AJNR Am J Neuroradiol 2011;32(1):34–40.
3. Molyneux AJ, Kerr RS, Yu LM, et al, International Subarachnoid Aneurysm Trial (ISAT) Collaborative Group. International Subarachnoid Aneurysm Trial (ISAT) of neurosurgical clipping versus endovascular coiling in 2143 patients with ruptured intracranial aneurysms: a randomised comparison of effects on survival, dependency, seizures, rebleeding, subgroups, and aneurysm occlusion. Lancet 2005;366:809–17.
4. Madaelil TP, Moran CJ, Cross DT 3rd, et al. Flow diversion in ruptured intracranial aneurysms: a meta-analysis. AJNR Am J Neuroradiol 2017;38:590–5.
5. Cagnazzo F, di Carlo DT, Cappucci M, et al. Acutely ruptured intracranial aneurysms treated with flow-diverter stents: a systematic review and meta-analysis. AJNR Am J Neuroradiol 2018;39:1669–75.

6. Hudson JS, Prout BS, Nagahama Y, et al. External ventricular drain and hemorrhage in aneurysmal subarachnoid hemorrhage patients on dual antiplatelet therapy: a retrospective cohort study. Neurosurgery 2019;84(2):479–84.

7. Hudson JS, Nagahama Y, Nakagawa D, et al. Hemorrhage associated with ventriculoperitoneal shunt placement in aneurysmal subarachnoid hemorrhage patients on a regimen of dual antiplatelet therapy: a retrospective analysis. J Neurosurg 2018;129(4): 916–21.

8. Girdhar G, Ubl S, Jahanbekam R, et al. Thrombogenicity assessment of pipeline, pipeline shield, Derivo and P64 flow diverters in an in vitro pulsatile flow human blood loop model. eNeurologicalSci 2019;14: 77–84. https://doi.org/10.1016/j.ensci.2019.01.004.

9. Trivelato FP, Wajnberg E, Rezende MT. Safety and effectiveness of the pipeline flex embolization device with shield technology for the treatement of Intracranial aneurysms: midterm results from a multicenter study. Neurosurgery 2020;87(1):104–11.

10. Galdamez MM, Lamin SM, Lagioes KG. Treatment of intracranial aneurysms using the pipeline flex embolization device with shield technology: angiographic and safety outcomes at 1-year follow up. J Neurointerv Surg 2019;11(4):396–9.

11. Pikis S, Mantziaris G, Mamalis V, et al. Diffusion weighted image documented cerebral ischemia in the post procedural period following pipeline embolization device with shield technology treatment of unruptured intracranial aneurysms: a prospective, single center study. J Neurointerv Surg 2020;12(4): 407–11.

12. Taschner C, Stracke CP, Dorn F, et al. Derivo embolization device in the treatment of unruptured intracranial aneurysms: a prospective multi center study. J Neurointerv Surg 2021;13(6):541–6.

13. Trvelato FP, Abud DG, Ulhoa AC, et al. Derivo embolization device for the treatment of intracranial aneurysms. Stroke 2019;50(9):2351–8.

14. Pierot L, Soize S, Cappucci M, et al. Surface-modified flow diverter p48-MW-HPC:preliminary clinical experience in 28 patients treated with two centers. J Neuroradiol 2021;48(3):195–9.

15. Schumacher AL, Gilmer CM, Atluri K, et al. Development and evaluation of a nanometer scale hemocompatible and antithrombotic coating technology platform for commercial intracranial stents and flow diverters. ACS Appl Nano Mater 2018;1(1):344–54.

16. Strelnikov N, Berestov V, Gorbatykh A, et al. Acute thrombus formation on phosphorilcholine surface modified flow diverters. Interv Neuroradiol 2018; 10(4):406–11.

17. Brinjikiji W, Lanzino G, Cloft HJ, et al. Rosk factors for ischemic complications following pipeline embolization device treatement of intreacranial aneurysms: results from the IntrePED Study. AJNR Am J Neuroradiol 2016;37(9):1673–8.

18. Becske T, Kallmes D, Saatci I, et al. Pipeline for uncoilable or failed aneurysms: results from a multicenter clinical trial. Radiology 2013;267(3):858–68.

19. Li Y-L, Roalfe A, Chu EY-L, et al. Outcome of flow diverters with surface modifications in treatment of cerebral aneurysms: systematic review and meta-analysis. AJNR Am J Neuroradiol 2021;42(2): 327–33.

20. Guzzardi G, Galbiati A, Stanca C, et al. Flow diverter stents with hydrophilic polymer coating for the treatment of ruptured intracranial aneurysms using single antiplatleet therapy; preliminary experience. Interv Neuroradiol 2021;26(5):525–31.

21. De Castro-Alfonso LH, Nakiri GS, Abud TG, et al. Aspirin monotherpay in the treatment of distal intracranial aneurysms with a surface modified flow diverter: a pilot study. J Neurointerv Surg 2021; 13(4):336–41.

22. Hanel RA, Aguilar-Salinas P, Brasiliense LB, et al. First US experience with pipeline flex with shield technology using aspirin as antiplatlet monotherapy. BMJ Case Rep 2017;2017. bcr2017219406.

23. Manning NW, Cheung A, Phillips TJ, et al. Pipeline shield with single antiplatlet therapy in aneurysmal subarachnoid hemorrhage: multicenter experience. J Neurointerv Surg 2019;11(7):694–8.

Advances in Intraarterial Chemotherapy Delivery Strategies and Blood-Brain Barrier Disruption

Kutluay Uluc, MD[a], Edward A. Neuwelt, MD[b,c,d], Prakash Ambady, MD[b],*

KEYWORDS

• Brain tumor • Chemotherapy • Intraarterial

KEY POINTS

- Although promising targeted agents show excellent in-vitro antitumor effects, clinical translation is frequently impeded due to a formidable physiologic barrier called the blood-brain barrier (BBB).
- Intraarterial route of delivery (IA) with osmotic blood-brain barrier disruption (BBBD) significantly increases drug concentration in the CNS compared to intravenous routes.
- In view of the excellent safety data and promising early efficacy data, IA/OBBBD warrents further evalutaion in multi-center prospective clinical trials.

INTRODUCTION

Incidence of primary brain tumors in the United States is estimated to be 24 per 100,000 persons.[1] Metastatic brain tumors are 10 times more common, and the incidence is expected to increase because better responses to new treatments of the primary disease are leading to longer survival.[2–4] Therapies for the treatment of primary or metastatic brain tumors remain a major challenge.[5] Surgical resection may be used as the sole therapy for benign and well-circumscribed lesions.[6] After maximal safe resection, however, chemotherapy and/or radiation therapy may be reserved for residual malignancy. These techniques are helpful to improve the overall survival and progression-free survival in the patients but are far from perfect. Although promising targeted agents show excellent in vitro antitumor effects, clinical translation is frequently impeded due to a formidable physiologic barrier called the blood-brain barrier (BBB). The BBB is composed of neurovascular units, which include endothelial tight junctions, astrocyte foot plates, basement membranes, and pericytes. Less than 2% of currently approved small-molecule drugs cross the BBB with an acceptable safety profile.[7] Accounting for first pass metabolism with traditional routes of chemotherapy delivery, significantly higher doses need to be used to have a reasonable therapeutic impact on the central nervous system (CNS), often leading to systemic toxicity.[8,9]

Intraarterial (IA) delivery bypasses the first pass effect/metabolism and has been used in several systemic cancers.[10–12] Furthermore, because this approach bypasses the first pass metabolism, IA delivery may allow the use of significantly lower chemotherapy doses and thus limit chemotherapy-related systemic toxicity. In animal models, a 2- to 5-fold increase in the drug concentration was observed with IA chemotherapy (IAC) when compared with standard intravenous (IV) chemotherapy doses.[13,14] IA delivery is not necessary for all chemotherapy agents, though. Especially chemotherapeutic agents with small molecular size, such as temozolomide, have

a Neurosurgery, Northernlight Eastern Maine Medical Center, Bangor, ME, USA; b Department of Neurology, Oregon Health & Science University, Portland, OR, USA; c Department of Neurosurgery, Oregon Health & Science University, Portland, OR, USA; d Portland Veterans Affairs Medical Center, Portland, OR, USA
* Corresponding author. Oregon Health Sciences University, L603 3181 SW Sam Jackson Park Road, Portland, OR 97239.
E-mail address: ambady@ohsu.edu

Neurosurg Clin N Am 33 (2022) 219–223
https://doi.org/10.1016/j.nec.2022.01.001

good CNS bioavailability when administered orally. IA administration of these agents may result in significantly increased drug concentration in the CNS and may therefore have unexpected side effects.[15] For large-molecule chemotherapeutic agents, however, disruption of the BBB would overcome the final obstacle to obtaining adequate concentrations for treatment.[13,16]

In this article, we review the history of IA drug delivery and osmotic blood-brain barrier disruption (OBBBD) and explore future directions.

HISTORY AND CURRENT STATUS

History of drug delivery to brain tumors cannot be discussed without discussing the BBB. The term blood-brain barrier was coined by Stern and Gautier in 1918.[17] IV chemotherapy has been used for the treatment of tumors since the late 1940s. Promising results were achieved initially in the treatment of Hodgkin disease, which expanded the use of chemotherapy for other pathologies.[18,19] Klopp and colleagues described the first use of IAC in animal models in 1950, followed by French and colleagues, who described the therapy in humans in 1952.[18] In 1972 Rapoport described the first BBBD by using an osmotic agent, mannitol/urea, the effects of which were reversible[20]; this was followed by our group describing IA delivery of mannitol for unlocking the BBB in 1979, later on in a clinical study in 1981.[21,22] Mohri and colleagues described use of IA delivery of melphalan, an ʟ-phenylalanine mustard, by using a balloon occlusion technique of internal carotid artery for the treatment of retinoblastoma in 1993.[18] Abramson and colleagues have improved on this technique by introducing selective catheterization of the ophthalmic artery in 2008.[10]

Significant success has been achieved in the management of retinoblastoma using IAC for multiple reasons. Even though the BBB and the blood-retinal barrier are similar, the BBB is 4 times more permeable to lipophilic substances, which may explain the success of IAC in retinoblastoma. It is thought that retinoblastoma may be more sensitive to chemotherapy when compared with brain tumors.[18]

Our group has a long experience of using the IA route for delivery of different chemotherapy agents, including carboplatin, temozolomide, melphalan, and methotrexate. Our experience in delivering these medications via the IA route have been published in many articles previously.[15,23–30] IA administration of other anticancer agents such as bevacizumab[31] and cetuximab[31] in conjunction with OBBBD has also been described by other groups.

Consideration of the BBB is a vital part of drug delivery, especially for large-molecule chemotherapy agents. One cannot overemphasize the importance of unlocking the BBB, and the use of osmotic agents is not the only technique for disrupting the BBB. Laser interstitial thermal therapy, ionizing radiation, MRI-guided focused ultrasound, convection enhanced delivery, and nanoparticle-based therapies all have been described to disrupt the BBB as well.[31–34]

IA delivery of methotrexate with adjunct OBBBD has resulted in durable tumor control and outcomes that are comparable or superior to other primary CNS lymphoma treatment regimens.[23] In 2000, a large multicenter study including approximately 2500 cases evaluated the safety of IA chemotherapy with BBBD in patients with various brain tumors. This study demonstrated a low incidence of catheter-related complications and enhanced delivery results with a high degree of tumor response. This efficacy profile was reproduced across multiple centers.[24] There are several rare complications associated with IA chemotherapy and OBBBD that have also been reported by our group, including cervical cord injury,[35] temozolomide-related toxicity,[15] and OBBBD-associated maculopathy.[36] Promising results for decreasing carboplatin-associated ototoxicity after IA with OBBBD were reported with the addition of sodium thiosulfate.[37]

Depending on the aggressiveness of the tumor, superselective IAC may be preferable over traditional IAC, and several studies have investigated this approach with promising results.[17] In 2011, Boockvar and colleagues reported treating 30 patients using bevacizumab with osmotic BBD. They demonstrated a good safety profile with nearly a 50% response in bevacizumab-naïve patients and a 15% response in patients who had previously received systemic bevacizumab.[31] In 2016, Chakraborty reported no procedural-related complications in their study in which cetuximab with osmotic BBBD was used for recurrent glioblastoma multiforme (GBM).[31,38]

TECHNICAL DETAILS OF INTRAARTERIAL DELIVERY

IA delivery is performed under conscious sedation (monitored anesthesia care) once every 4 weeks. In these treatment sessions, the whole cerebral circulation is treated with slight alterations depending on the vascular anatomy.

Access to the right femoral artery is achieved with a 19-gauge needle and a 5-French diagnostic catheter introduced using Seldinger technique. The left internal carotid artery (LICA) at C1-2 level, right internal carotid artery (RICA) at C1-2 level, and, depending on anatomy, either the right vertebral artery (RVA) or left vertebral artery (LVA) at C4-5 level are selectively catheterized. Chemotherapy is then given. After the procedure, patients are transferred to the general care floor for monitoring of vital signs, neurologic status, and fluid balance. They are generally discharged the day following the procedure.

TECHNICAL DETAILS OF INTRAARTERIAL DELIVERY WITH OSMOTIC BLOOD-BRAIN BARRIER DISRUPTION

OBBBD is performed under generalized anesthesia with propofol because this may be painful for the patient. Avoidance of other anesthetics is important to improve the BBB opening. The patient receives therapy on 2 consecutive days every 4 weeks up to 1 year or 12 cycles.

Before the treatment, patients are hydrated with D5 1/2NS at 100 to 150 mL/h for a minimum of 6 hours. Patients are premedicated with an anticonvulsant (commonly levetiracetam), for postoperative seizure risk. OBBBD may cause bradycardia; therefore, atropine is administered IV immediately before mannitol administration.

Selective arterial catheterization is performed depending on the cerebral vascular territory (LICA vs RICA vs RVA vs LVA) that is planned to be treated after femoral access is achieved as described earlier. One territory per day is treated. To perform OBBBD, warm (37° C) 25% mannitol is administered at 4 to 10 mL/s (precise flow rate is determined by use of fluoroscopy) for 30 seconds. A nonionic

contrast agent (750 mbq of Tc-99m glucoheptonate and 150 mL Isovue-300 iopamidol)[39] is administered IV after OBBBD, and a computed tomography (CT) brain scan (**Fig. 1**) is obtained for evaluation of the degree of disruption. For documentation of the degree of disruption, contrast enhancement in the disrupted territory is compared with nondisrupted territory by visual grading of the CT. Four grades are used: nil, moderate, good, or excellent. Diuretics or fluid boluses are used in management of fluid balance. After the procedure, patients are transferred to the postanesthesia care unit and then the general care floor for monitoring of vital signs, neurologic status, and fluid balance.

FUTURE DIRECTIONS

There are reports of using pulsatile injection[40] or slower infusion rates[41] to improve drug concentrations and minimize toxicity; there is, however, no consensus on optimal rate and type of injection/infusion. Future studies comparing the optimal rate of injection/infusion and type of infusion are necessary to find the ideal delivery method.

With emerging catheter technology and endovascular techniques, complication rates are decreasing further, which is enabling more targeted therapies. The benefits of superselective therapy include avoiding some complications such as cervical cord injury,[35] chemotherapy-related toxicity,[15] OBBBD-associated maculopathy,[36] and

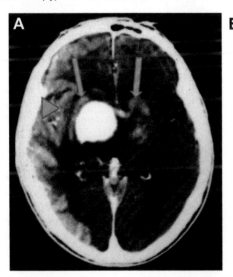 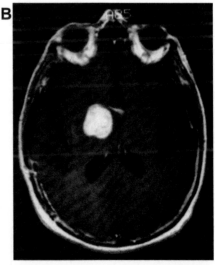

Fig. 1. Contrast-enhanced CT scan allows quantification of the degree of disruption after OBBBD. (*A*) Gadolinium-enhanced T1-weighted MRI demonstrates avidly enhancing parenchymal lesion. (*B*) Contrast-enhanced CT scan, post-OBBBD via right internal carotid artery. A CT-based visual scale (0 = no disruption, 1 = moderate, 2 = good, and 3 = excellent disruption) was developed and validated by the Neuwelt laboratory to quantify the degree of disruption[39]. As expected, areas with higher vascularity such as the cortex demonstrate a greater degree of disruption (*blue arrowhead*). In addition, contrast enhancement is now evident in the previously nonenhancing brain around the tumor (*blue arrow*) after OBBBD. IA with OBBBD allows the use of the unique anatomy of the circle of Willis and allows regional disruption and better drug delivery to the infiltrating tumor edge and the brain around the tumor. This case would be graded 3 (excellent disruption).

carboplatin-associated ototoxicity.[37] Careful evaluation of disease progression should be done when making decisions about treating a specific arterial distribution or the whole brain because widespread diseases such as GBM may recur in distant locations. Treating a selective distribution of these types of cancers may therefore result in adequate treatment. Superselective treatment should be compared with traditional IAC, especially for widespread pathologies such as metastatic brain tumors and malignant brain tumors.

A recent study demonstrated that OBBBD using mannitol generates a transient sterile neuroinflammatory response marked by increased production of cytokines, chemokines, and trophic factors, leading to activation of astrocytes, microglia, and macrophages.[42] With promising results and recent advances in immunotherapy for hematological and solid malignancies,[43] this finding may open a new frontier for the use of immunotherapy in the treatment of brain tumors via OBBBD.

Although this procedure is well tolerated by patients, currently, OBBBD can only be performed at select centers. Concerted collaborative efforts to standardize and optimize this technique needs to be an important focus to enable generalizability. In addition, detailed and long-term neurocognitive, ocular, and ototoxicity evaluation needs to be included in all future studies in addition to patient's quality of life and satisfaction scores.

SUMMARY

IA chemotherapy delivery has several advantages compared with IV delivery. These advantages can further be augmented by addition of BBBD. Further understanding the tumor biology, pathophysiology, and the effect of the microenvironment is going to shape future strategies for administration of chemotherapy. In view of the excellent safety data and promising early efficacy data, IAC combined with OBBBD needs to be a considered in addition to traditional approaches when new CNS-targeted agents are being evaluated in clinical trials.

CLINICS CARE POINTS

- Intraarterial route of delivery (IA) with osmotic blood-brain barrier disruption (BBBD) can significantly increases drug concentration in the CNS compared to intravenous routes.
- In view of the excellent safety data and promising early efficacy data, IA/OBBBD warrents further evaluation in multi-center prospective clinical trials.

REFERENCES

1. Ostrom QT, Patil N, Cioffi G, et al. CBTRUS Statistical Report: Primary Brain and Other Central Nervous System Tumors Diagnosed in the United States in 2013-2017. Neuro Oncol 2020;22(12 Suppl 2):iv1–96.
2. Johnson JD, Young B. Demographics of brain metastasis. Neurosurg Clin N Am 1996;7(3):337–44.
3. Wen PY, Loeffler JS. Management of brain metastases. Oncol (Williston Park) 1999;13(7):941–54, 957-954.
4. Hádlík J, Sindelárová M, Svestka J. [Experimental and clinical experiences with Encephabol therapy in gerontopsychiatry]. Cesk Psychiatr 1971;67(3):129–33.
5. Perkins A, Liu G. Primary Brain Tumors in Adults: Diagnosis and Treatment. Am Fam Physician 2016; 93(3):211–7.
6. Aghi M, Barker Ii FG. Benign adult brain tumors: an evidence-based medicine review. Prog Neurol Surg 2006;19:80–96.
7. Pardridge WM. The blood-brain barrier: bottleneck in brain drug development. Neurorx 2005;2(1):3–14.
8. Pond SM, Tozer TN. First-pass elimination. Basic concepts and clinical consequences. Clin Pharm 1984;9(1):1–25.
9. Wang Z, Sun H, Yakisich JS. Overcoming the blood-brain barrier for chemotherapy: limitations, challenges and rising problems. Anticancer Agents Med Chem 2014;14(8):1085–93.
10. Abramson DH, Dunkel IJ, Brodie SE, et al. A phase I/II study of direct intraarterial (ophthalmic artery) chemotherapy with melphalan for intraocular retinoblastoma initial results. Ophthalmol 2008;115(8): 1398–404, 1404.e1.
11. Fortin D, Gendron C, Boudrias M, et al. Enhanced chemotherapy delivery by intraarterial infusion and blood-brain barrier disruption in the treatment of cerebral metastasis. Cancer 2007;109(4):751–60.
12. Dumortier J, Decullier E, Hilleret MN, et al. Adjuvant Intraarterial Lipiodol or ^{131}I-Lipiodol After Curative Treatment of Hepatocellular Carcinoma: A Prospective Randomized Trial. J Nucl Med 2014;55(6):877–83.
13. Neuwelt EA, Barnett PA, Frenkel EP. Chemotherapeutic agent permeability to normal brain and delivery to avian sarcoma virus-induced brain tumors in the rodent: observations on problems of drug delivery. Neurosurg 1984;14(2):154–60.
14. Kroll RA, Neuwelt EA. Outwitting the blood-brain barrier for therapeutic purposes: osmotic opening and other means. Neurosurg 1998;42(5):1083–99.
15. Muldoon LL, Pagel MA, Netto JP, et al. Intra-arterial administration improves temozolomide delivery and efficacy in a model of intracerebral metastasis, but has unexpected brain toxicity. J Neurooncol 2016; 126(3):447–54.
16. Neuwelt EA, Minna J, Frenkel E, et al. Osmotic blood-brain barrier opening to IgM monoclonal antibody in the rat. Am J Phys 1986;250(5 Pt 2):R875–83.

17. Saunders NR, Dreifuss JJ, Dziegielewska KM, et al. The rights and wrongs of blood-brain barrier permeability studies: a walk through 100 years of history. Front Neurosci 2014;8:404.

18. Srinivasan VM, Lang FF, Chen SR, et al. Advances in endovascular neuro-oncology: endovascular selective intra-arterial (ESIA) infusion of targeted biologic therapy for brain tumors. J Neurointerv Surg 2020; 12(2):197–203.

19. Sawyer AJ, Piepmeier JM, Saltzman WM. New methods for direct delivery of chemotherapy for treating brain tumors. Yale J Biol Med 2006;79(3–4):141–52.

20. Rapoport SI, Hori M, Klatzo I. Testing of a hypothesis for osmotic opening of the blood-brain barrier. Am J Physiol 1972;223(2):323–31.

21. Neuwelt EA, Frenkel EP, Diehl JT, et al. Osmotic blood-brain barrier disruption: a new means of increasing chemotherapeutic agent delivery. Trans Am Neurol Assoc 1979;104:256–60.

22. Neuwelt EA, Hill SA, Frenkel EP, et al. Osmotic blood-brain barrier disruption: pharmacodynamic studies in dogs and a clinical phase I trial in patients with malignant brain tumors. Cancer Treat Rep 1981; 65(Suppl 2):39–43.

23. Angelov L, Doolittle ND, Kraemer DF, et al. Blood-brain barrier disruption and intra-arterial methotrexate-based therapy for newly diagnosed primary CNS lymphoma: a multi-institutional experience. J Clin Oncol 2009;27(21):3503–9.

24. Doolittle ND, Miner ME, Hall WA, et al. Safety and efficacy of a multicenter study using intraarterial chemotherapy in conjunction with osmotic opening of the blood-brain barrier for the treatment of patients with malignant brain tumors. Cancer 2000;88(3):637–47.

25. Guillaume DJ, Doolittle ND, Gahramanov S, et al. Intraarterial chemotherapy with osmotic blood-brain barrier disruption for aggressive oligodendroglial tumors: results of a phase I study. Neurosurg 2010;66(1):48–58.

26. Doolittle ND, Muldoon LL, Culp AY, et al. Delivery of chemotherapeutics across the blood-brain barrier: challenges and advances. Adv Pharmacol 2014;71:203–43.

27. Jahnke K, Kraemer DF, Knight KR, et al. Intraarterial chemotherapy and osmotic blood-brain barrier disruption for patients with embryonal and germ cell tumors of the central nervous system. Cancer 2008;112(3):581–8.

28. Uluc K, Siler DA, Lopez R, et al. Long-Term Outcomes of Intra-Arterial Chemotherapy for Progressive or Unresectable Pilocytic Astrocytomas: Case Studies. Neurosurgery 2021;88(4):E336–42.

29. Osztie E, Várallyay P, Doolittle ND, et al. Combined intraarterial carboplatin, intraarterial etoposide phosphate, and IV Cytoxan chemotherapy for progressive optic-hypothalamic gliomas in young children. AJNR Am J Neuroradiol 2001;22(5):818–23.

30. Hall WA, Doolittle ND, Daman M, et al. Osmotic blood-brain barrier disruption chemotherapy for diffuse pontine gliomas. J Neurooncol 2006;77(3):279–84.

31. Boockvar JA, Tsiouris AJ, Hofstetter CP, et al. Safety and maximum tolerated dose of superselective intraarterial cerebral infusion of bevacizumab after osmotic blood-brain barrier disruption for recurrent malignant glioma. Clin article. J Neurosurg 2011;114(3):624–32.

32. D'Amico RS, Khatri D, Reichman N, et al. Super selective intra-arterial cerebral infusion of modern chemotherapeutics after blood-brain barrier disruption: where are we now, and where are we going. J Neurooncol 2020;147(2):261–78.

33. Li YQ, Chen P, Haimovitz-Friedman A, et al. Endothelial apoptosis initiates acute blood-brain barrier disruption after ionizing radiation. Cancer Res 2003;63(18):5950–6.

34. Hendricks BK, Cohen-Gadol AA, Miller JC. Novel delivery methods bypassing the blood-brain and blood-tumor barriers. Neurosurg Focus 2015;38(3):E10.

35. Fortin D, McAllister LD, Nesbit G, et al. Unusual cervical spinal cord toxicity associated with intra-arterial carboplatin, intra-arterial or intravenous etoposide phosphate, and intravenous cyclophosphamide in conjunction with osmotic blood brain-barrier disruption in the vertebral artery. AJNR Am J Neuroradiol 1999;20(10):1794–802.

36. Simonett JM, Skalet AH, Lujan BJ, et al. Risk Factors and Disease Course for Blood-Brain Barrier Disruption-Associated Maculopathy. JAMA Ophthalmol 2021;139(2):143–9.

37. Neuwelt EA, Gilmer-Knight K, Lacy C, et al. Toxicity profile of delayed high dose sodium thiosulfate in children treated with carboplatin in conjunction with blood-brain-barrier disruption. Pediatr Blood Cancer 2006;47(2):174–82.

38. Chakraborty S, Filippi CG, Wong T, et al. Superselective intraarterial cerebral infusion of cetuximab after osmotic blood/brain barrier disruption for recurrent malignant glioma: phase I study. J Neurooncol 2016;128(3):405–15.

39. Roman-Goldstein S, Clunie DA, Stevens J, et al. Osmotic blood-brain barrier disruption: CT and radionuclide imaging. AJNR Am J Neuroradiol 1994;15(3):581–90.

40. Gobin YP, Cloughesy TF, Chow KL, et al. Intraarterial chemotherapy for brain tumors by using a spatial dose fractionation algorithm and pulsatile delivery. Radiol 2001;218(3):724–32.

41. Blacklock JB, Wright DC, Dedrick RL, et al. Drug streaming during intra-arterial chemotherapy. J Neurosurg 1986;64(2):284–91.

42. Burks SR, Kersch CN, Witko JA, et al. Blood-brain barrier opening by intracarotid artery hyperosmolar mannitol induces sterile inflammatory and innate immune responses. Proc Natl Acad Sci U S A 2021;(18):118.

43. Kruger S, Ilmer M, Kobold S, et al. Advances in cancer immunotherapy 2019 - latest trends. J Exp Clin Cancer Res 2019;38(1):268.

Endovascular Robotic Interventions

Kareem El Naamani, MD, Rawad Abbas, MD, Georgios S. Sioutas, MD,
Stavropoula I. Tjoumakaris, MD, Michael R. Gooch, MD, Nabeel A. Herial, MD, MPH,
Robert H. Rosenwasser, MD, MBA, Pascal M. Jabbour, MD*

KEYWORDS

• Carotid angioplasty stenting • Robotic-assisted • Technology • Peripheral vascular interventions

KEY POINTS

• The CorPath GRX Robotic System received Food and Drug Administration approval for peripheral vascular interventions in 2018.
• Robotic assistance dramatically reduces the amount of radiation exposure and the rate of orthopedic injuries.
• The most important advantage of robotic assistance is the ability to perform remote procedures.
• The main disadvantage of robotic assistance is the absence of haptic feedback.

 Video content accompanies this article at http://www.neurosurgery.theclinics.com.

INTRODUCTION

Over the past 2 decades, technological advancements in robotics have revolutionized surgical procedures. Early models have been used in several surgical specialties, but it was not until a few years ago that robotic systems reached the endovascular neurosurgery field.[1] The purpose of incorporating robots in surgical technique is to maximize consistency, dexterity, remote access, and human performance beyond intrinsic physical limitations while minimizing occupational hazards and human error.[2] After receiving Food and Drug Administration (FDA) approval in 2016 for percutaneous coronary interventions (PCI) and in 2018 for peripheral vascular interventions (PVI), the CorPath GRX Robotic System (Corindus Inc, Waltham, MA, USA) has been incorporated in the endovascular neurosurgical field, mainly in treating carotid artery diseases.[3] The use of robotic systems in endovascular neurosurgery is still in its infancy. With the high level of precision and speed the field requires, however, robotic systems could play a pivotal role in providing increased levels of care. Corpath GRX has been introduced in several centers across the globe and is being used in carotid angioplasty stenting and other endovascular procedures. Herein, we will summarize the literature pertaining to our current experience with robotic systems and delineate the progress of future directions.

History of Robotic Systems

Since Moniz first used radiopaque dye and radiography to visualize cerebral vessels in 1927, major technological advancements have been achieved in the field of endovascular interventions in treating aneurysms, vascular malformations, strokes, subdural hematomas, and other pathologies.[4,5]

Funding statement: This research received no specific grant from any funding agency in public, commercial, or not-for-profit sectors.
Department of Neurological Surgery, Thomas Jefferson University Hospital, 901 Walnut Street 3rd Floor, Philadelphia, PA 19107, USA
* Corresponding author.
E-mail address: pascal.jabbour@jefferson.edu

Neurosurg Clin N Am 33 (2022) 225–231
https://doi.org/10.1016/j.nec.2021.11.008
1042-3680/22/© 2021 Elsevier Inc. All rights reserved.

Despite this progress, these procedures require an operator to stand table-side in the interventional neuroradiology suite and manually inject contrast and manipulate wires and catheters, all while being exposed to radiation. The first experience with a robotic surgical system started in 1983 with Arthrobot, which was used to aid orthopedic surgeries in Canada.[6] Several experimental robotic systems followed, but it was not until the introduction of the da Vinci surgical robotic system (Intuitive Surgical) in 2000 that significant steps were noted in the fields of urology, gynecology, and head and neck surgery.[7] In 2007 the Sensei robotic system was FDA approved for ablative cardiac procedures.[8] In 2013, the Percutaneous Robotically Enhanced Coronary Intervention Study (PRECISE) pivotal trial demonstrated the safety, efficacy, and feasibility of robotic-assisted PCI using the CorPath 200 (Corindus Inc., Waltham, USA).[9] Because of this, use of robotic systems gained interest in the endovascular neurointerventional field, and the CorPath GRX Robotic System (Corindus Inc, Waltham, MA, USA) was FDA approved for PCI procedures in 2016 and PVI procedures in 2018.[3]

Set-Up

Endovascular robotic systems consist of 2 main components: the patient-side robot and the control station[5] (**Fig. 1**). Since the control station is equipped with a radiation-shielded cockpit, it is usually present in the procedure room. However, in other set-ups, the control station is situated outside the procedure room, which eliminates radiation exposure for the physician.[1,5,10] The control-station is composed of several screens, sensors, and joysticks to control the bed-side robot. Fluoroscopy and hemodynamic monitors enable real-time visualization.[1,5] Instructions are sent from the control station to the patient-side robot, which in turn physically manipulates the endovascular catheters and wires.[5] The bed-side robot consists of an articulated arm, a robotic drive, and a disposable cassette[1] (**Figs. 2** and **3**). The cassette is responsible for translating real-time commands from the control station, which enables the physicians to manipulate the robotic arm using the joysticks.[10] The robotic system is compatible with 0.014 and 0.018 inch guidewires, rapid exchange catheters, and several other devices that can be manipulated with one hand, allowing the operation of an automatic contrast media injector with the other.[1] Extremely precise movements can be performed using the joysticks while movement of the devices is observed on the fluoroscopy monitor.

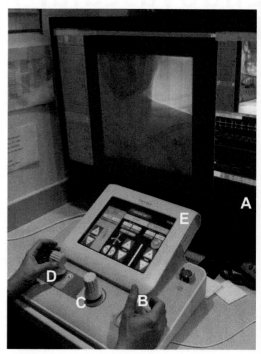

Fig. 1. Control station of the robotic system. (A) High-definition screen to view fluoroscopy images; (B) guide catheter/diagnostic catheter joystick; (C) guide-wire joystick; (D) device joystick; (E) joystick feedback monitor.

When a procedure takes place, the robotic arm is covered with sterile drapes and the cassette is attached to the platform of the arm. When the physician decides which catheter will be used, the proximal part of the catheter is attached to the hemostatic valve (Copilot, Santa Clara,

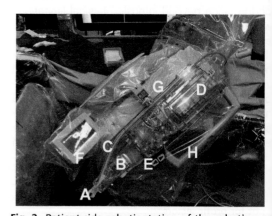

Fig. 2. Patient-side robotic station of the robotic system. (A) Sheath attachment; (B) guide catheter rotation module; (C) guide support track; (D) guide wire rotation module; (E) microadjustment buttons; (F) robotic arm feedback console; (G) cassette lock (*yellow arrow*); (H) robotic arm toggle button.

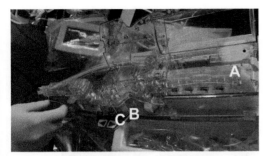

Fig. 3. Cassette shown open. (A) disposable cassette; (B) device port (*orange arrow*); (C) manual port (*orange arrow*).

California, USA) and secured to the guide slot of the cassette along with the copilot.[1] After that, the guide support track is pulled over the catheter and locked onto the side port of the radial sheath (**Fig. 4**). Then the cassette is locked, and the robotic unit is ready to manipulate the catheter. It only takes 20 sec to install a new device into the cassette.[1] When set-up is completed, the access site is punctured manually and the catheter is advanced based on which procedure is taking place.[1] At this point, the catheter is connected to the robotic arm and the physician takes over the procedure at the control station (**Fig. 5**).(Video 1).

Advantages

Robotic systems provide several advantages to both patients and physicians. With respect to patients, physiologic tremor of the operator is eliminated potentially allowing safer navigation, more precise device control, and smoother deployment.[1] The robot's steady arms deliver exception precision beyond even the most skilled and experience human hands for long hours without any fatigue or decrease in efficiency.[2] Moreover, the incorporation of artificial intelligence algorithms in

these robotic systems leads to constant evolution and better consistence among operators.[2] As for physicians, robotic assistance brings several advantages related to occupational hazards. According to Roguin and colleagues, out of 31 brain tumors collected from physicians exposed to ionizing radiation, 85% are left-sided brain tumors and most of the physicians were interventional cardiologists.[11] These data were supported by the Brain Radioactive Exposure and Attenuation During Invasive Cardiology Procedures (BRAIN) trial, which showed that not only is radiation exposure higher on the left cranium during interventional cardiology procedures, but also the risk of these brain tumors will increase with the spread of transradial approaches.[12] Furthermore, a survey performed in the Society for Cardiovascular Angiography and Interventions showed that 50% of the responders suffer from at least one orthopedic problem.[13] Although these studies were done in the cardiology field, they reflect the problems faced in the neurointerventional field, as both fields have the same working environment. Also, according to the Retrospective Evaluation study of Lens Injuries and Dose (RELID), interventionalists have cataract-type eye opacities 3 times more often compared with an age-matched control group.[14] Thus, by allowing the physicians to sit comfortably without lead apron wear in a protected environment, robotic assistance dramatically reduces the amount of radiation exposure and the rate of orthopedic injuries.[1,2,15] In addition, it has been proved that the learning curve for a Corindus robot is short and by performing 3 cases, interventionalists become quicker and more efficient in completing robotic-assisted procedures.[9] Perhaps, the most important advantage of robotic assistance is the ability to perform remote procedures. Although remote procedures have been done for cardiac PCIs, this feature will be pivotal in treating strokes in low-resource or remote areas

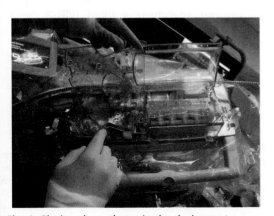

Fig. 4. Placing the catheter in the device port.

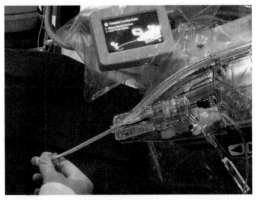

Fig. 5. Connecting the catheter to the robotic arm.

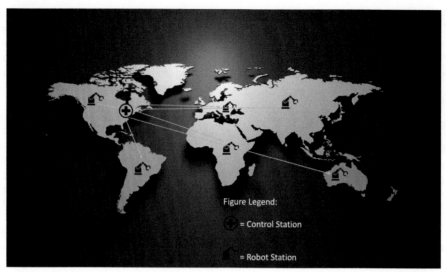

Fig. 6. Telerobotic stroke system. A neurointerventionalist can control remote robotic systems to expand the network of care.

when intracranial robotic procedures become FDA approved[16,17] (**Fig. 6**).

Disadvantages

Despite the overall promising results, it is essential to remember that these robotic systems have been developed for PCIs and PVIs, and currently they lack the ability to perform more complex intracranial procedures.[2] Also, in the current approved procedures, the physician or a trained representative still needs to obtain vascular access. Other personnel are still needed in the room to operate the table. The main disadvantage is the absence of haptic feedback, which neurointerventionalists heavily rely on during microcatheter, microwire, and device manipulation in intracranial procedures.[18] Also, the inability of the cassette in the current robotic systems to manipulate over the wire equipment hinders the use of almost all modern neurointerventional devices.[1] An additional limitation is if these systems are to be FDA approved and used in remote procedures, they will require extremely high speeds of data transfer and possibly increase difficulty of salvage in cases of complications.[1] Moreover, these systems are expensive (about $600,000) and each disposable cassette costs $500.[1] Another concern is reimbursement and licensing in the relevant jurisdiction. Medicolegally, regulatory bodies approving the companies that provide robotic systems will mandate that an interventionalist be present on site to supervise and guide these interventions.[19] The remote nature of these procedures and the administrative complexity required to perform them between states and countries further complicate the medicolegal aspect especially in cases of complications and mortality. Lastly, as mentioned earlier, robotic systems are still in infancy, and there is a paucity of information about this emerging technology. Because of this, it is pivotal that more trials be performed to assess the learning curve, nature and rate of complications, and a noninferiority study to compare patient care, anesthesia, and postprocedural care between robotic systems and the conventional treatment modalities.

Literature Review

Several centers around the world have adopted robotic systems in their diagnostic and interventional procedures and have provided their experience with these systems. In 2016, Lu and colleagues reported no complications after using the vascular interventional robot (VIR-2; Navy General Hospital of People's Liberation Army, Beijing University) in 15 diagnostic cerebral angiographies.[20] In 2017, Vuong and colleagues shared their experience using the Magellan Robotic Catheter System (Hansen Medical) in 9 diagnostic cerebral angiographies.[6] Their study showed no significant difference in fluoroscopy time, contrast volume, and procedural time between robotic-assisted diagnostic angiographies and manual angiographies.[6] In 2019, Nogueira and colleagues reported successful completion of 4 cases of robotic-assisted carotid stenting without any complications using the CorPath GRX Robotic System.[2] In 2020, we published our experience with

Table 1
Summary of all the studies sharing their experience with robotic systems in endovascular neurointerventions

Study (Year)	Robot Name	Number of Patients	Diagnostic	Intervention	Complications
Lu et al,[20] 2016	Vascular Interventional Robot	15	15	0	None
Vuong et al,[6] 2017	Magellan Robotic Catheter System	9	9	0	None
Nogueira et al,[2] 2019	CorPath GRX Robotic System	4	0	Robotic-Assisted Carotid Stenting (n = 4)	None
Sajja et al,[1] 2020	CorPath GRX Robotic System	10	7	Robotic-Assisted Carotid Stenting (n = 3)	Converted to manual diagnostic angiographies because of bovine aortic arches
Weinberg et al,[3] 2020	CorPath GRX Robotic System	6	0	Robotic-Assisted Carotid Stenting (n = 6)	None
George et al,[21] 2020	CorPath GRX Robotic System	1	0	Robotic-Assisted Carotid Stenting (n = 1)	None
Pereira et al,[15] 2020	CorPath GRX Robotic System	1	0	Stent-Assisted Coiling (n = 1)	None

the CorPath GRX Robotic System. The robotic system was used in 7 diagnostic cerebral angiographies and 3 cases of robotic-assisted carotid angioplasty and stenting. All the planned technical steps were completed without complications except in 3 patients of the diagnostic group who had bovine aortic arches, which required conversion to manual.[1] Also, George and colleagues reported their successful experience in treating a patient via robotic-assisted carotid stenting with no complications after she was deemed a high-risk patient for carotid endarterectomy.[21] We also conducted a retrospective study in which we compared 6 robotic-assisted transradial carotid stenting procedures with manual carotid stenting in 2020. Our study showed significant longer procedure time in the robotic group but no significant difference between both modalities with respect to fluoroscopy time, contrast dose, radiation exposure, catheter exchange, technical success, transfemoral conversion, and complications.[3] Pereira and colleagues were granted off-label approve for the use of this robotic system for the first intracranial intervention. They were able to perform a stent-assisted coiling of a 12-mm basilar trunk aneurysm with no complications. On follow-up the patient had normal functional outcome, and the aneurysm was completely occluded.[5,15] These cases are summarized in **Table 1**. As for the learning curve, a recent study at our institution displayed similar results to the literature by showing that few robotics cases are enough to overcome the learning curve and significantly decrease procedure and fluoroscopy time.[1,22]

SUMMARY

With the introduction of robotic systems to the endovascular neurosurgical field, many centers have started experimenting the boundaries of this new technology. Although robotic systems are still not FDA approved for intracranial interventional procedures, the promising results these systems have shown in PCIs show the great potential that can be achieved in providing precise and consistent neurosurgical care in a way that offers minimized radiation exposure and improved ergonomics, with potential future applications to remote locations benefiting those patients living in remote geographic areas.

CLINICS CARE POINTS

- Robotic systems decrease the rate of radiation exposure because the interventionalist is performing the procedure in the radiation-shielded cockpit.
- Robotic systems have come a long way, but still require further advancements to perfect intracranial procedures.

COMPETING INTERESTS

Dr P.M. Jabbour is a consultant for Medtronic and MicroVention. Dr S.I. Tjoumakaris and Dr M.R. Gooch are consultants for Stryker. The other authors have no personal, financial, or institutional interest in any of the drugs, materials, or devices described in this article.

ACKNOWLEDGMENTS

None.

DISCLOSURE

This research received no specific grant from any funding agency in public, commercial, or not-for-profit sectors.

SUPPLEMENTARY DATA

Supplementary data related to this article can be found online at https://doi.org/10.1016/j.nec.2021.11.008.

REFERENCES

1. Sajja KC, Sweid A, Al Saiegh F, et al. Endovascular robotic: feasibility and proof of principle for diagnostic cerebral angiography and carotid artery stenting. J Neurointerv Surg 2020;12:345–9.
2. Nogueira RG, Sachdeva R, Al-Bayati AR, et al. Robotic assisted carotid artery stenting for the treatment of symptomatic carotid disease: technical feasibility and preliminary results. J Neurointerv Surg 2020;12:341–4.
3.. Weinberg JH, Sweid A, Sajja K, et al. Comparison of robotic-assisted carotid stenting and manual carotid stenting through the transradial approach. J Neurosurg 2020;135(1):1–8.
4. Moniz E. Arterial encephalography, its importance in the localization of cerebral tumors. J Neurosurg 1964;21:145–56.
5. Beaman CB, Kaneko N, Meyers PM, et al. A review of robotic interventional neuroradiology. Am J Neuroradiology 2021;42:808.
6. Vuong SM, Carroll CP, Tackla RD, et al. Application of emerging technologies to improve access to ischemic stroke care. Neurosurg Focus 2017;42:E8.
7. Yates DR, Vaessen C, Roupret M. From Leonardo to da Vinci: the history of robot-assisted surgery in urology. BJU Int 2011;108:1708–13 [discussion: 1714].
8. Bismuth J, Duran C, Stankovic M, et al. A first-in-man study of the role of flexible robotics in overcoming navigation challenges in the iliofemoral arteries. J Vasc Surg 2013;57:14s–9s.
9. Weisz G, Metzger DC, Caputo RP, et al. Safety and feasibility of robotic percutaneous coronary intervention: PRECISE (Percutaneous Robotically-Enhanced Coronary Intervention) Study. J Am Coll Cardiol 2013;61:1596–600.
10. Granada JF, Delgado JA, Uribe MP, et al. First-in-human evaluation of a novel robotic-assisted coronary angioplasty system. JACC Cardiovasc Interv 2011;4:460–5.
11. Roguin A, Goldstein J, Bar O, et al. Brain and neck tumors among physicians performing interventional procedures. Am J Cardiol 2013;111:1368–72.
12. Reeves RR, Ang L, Bahadorani J, et al. Invasive cardiologists are exposed to greater left sided cranial radiation: The BRAIN Study (brain radiation exposure and attenuation during invasive cardiology procedures). JACC Cardiovasc Interv 2015;8:1197–206.
13. Klein LW, Tra Y, Garratt KN, et al. Occupational health hazards of interventional cardiologists in the current decade: Results of the 2014 SCAI membership survey. Catheter Cardiovasc Interv 2015;86:913–24.
14. Papp C, Romano-Miller M, Descalzo A, et al. Results of Relid Study 2014-Buenos Aires, Argentina Retrospective Evaluation of Lens Injuries and Dose. Radiat Prot Dosimetry 2017;173:212–7.
15. Mendes Pereira V, Cancelliere NM, Nicholson P, et al. First-in-human, robotic-assisted neuroendovascular intervention. J Neurointerv Surg 2020;12:338–40.
16. Patel TM, Shah SC, Pancholy SB. Long distance tele-robotic-assisted percutaneous coronary intervention: a report of first-in-human experience. EClinicalMedicine 2019;14:53–8.
17. Madder RD, VanOosterhout S, Mulder A, et al. Feasibility of robotic telestenting over long geographic

distances: a pre-clinical ex vivo and in vivo study. EuroIntervention 2019;15:e510–2.

18. Da L, Zhang D, Wang T. Overview of the vascular interventional robot. Int J Med Robot 2008;4:289–94.

19. Goyal M, Sutherland GR, Lama S, et al. Neurointerventional robotics: challenges and opportunities. Clin Neuroradiology 2020;30:203–8.

20. Lu WS, Xu WY, Pan F, et al. Clinical application of a vascular interventional robot in cerebral angiography. Int J Med Robot 2016;12:132–6.

21. George JC, Tabaza L, Janzer S. Robotic-assisted balloon angioplasty and stent placement with distal embolic protection device for severe carotid artery stenosis in a high-risk surgical patient. Catheter Cardiovasc Interv 2020;96:410–2.

22. Weisz G, Smilowitz NR, Metzger DC, et al. The association between experience and proficiency with robotic-enhanced coronary intervention-insights from the PRECISE multi-center study. Acute Card Care 2014;16:37–40.

Future Directions of Endovascular Neurosurgery

Kurt Yaeger, MD*, J Mocco, MD, MS

KEYWORDS

- Brain–computer interface • Endovascular • Devices • Stent • Technology

KEY POINTS

- Endovascular neurosurgery has a rich history of device and technique innovation.
- Over the years, new endovascular strategies have facilitated the treatment of conditions without definitive therapy, such as ischemic stroke and chronic subdural hematoma.
- The Stentrode brain–computer interface is an endovascularly-deployed stent for recording neural signals, which can be converted to a motor output, and has been used in humans to facilitate ADLs.
- The eShunt is an endovascularly deployed shunt for idiopathic intracranial hypertension that creates a fistula between the cerebellopontine angle cistern and the inferior petrosal sinus that allows CSF to drain via the natural pressure gradient into the venous system.
- These innovations, in addition to novel devices for wide-neck aneurysms, highlight the future of endovascular neurosurgery in pushing the limit for treatable neuropathology.

BACKGROUND: A RICH HISTORY OF NEUROENDOVASCULAR INNOVATION

Endovascular Neurosurgery evolved predominantly as a means to treat cerebrovascular pathology. From Gugliemi detachable coils for intracranial aneurysms to liquid embolic agents for arteriovenous malformations (AVMs), early technical innovations in the field facilitated alternatives to open craniotomy and microneurosurgery. Yet, as a specialty limited by the available technology, pioneers in the field have continued innovating and expanding the range of cerebrovascular pathologies treatable by an endovascular approach. Furthermore, at the present time, we are witnessing the emergence of new neurologic disease states treated by endovascular techniques, driven by device innovation and constant technique refinement. We discuss the future of endovascular neurosurgery and the neurointerventionalist's role in expanding indications for previously untreatable conditions, as well as continuing to improve the safety and efficacy of existing techniques.

To best explore the future of endovascular neurosurgery, one must assess the rich history of technical innovation in the field. Before the early 2000s, ischemic stroke was a nonsurgical disease process, with only modest efficacy of the best medical management with systemic intravenous thrombolysis.[1] However, the persistence of neuro-interventionalists to surgically treat the mechanical obstruction of large vessel occlusions (LVOs) had led to one of the most profound paradigm shifts in modern medicine. After failing to see a major benefit with intra-arterial thrombolysis for acute ischemic stroke, interventionalists turned to devices for mechanical clot disruption.[2] Ultimately, investigating the MERCI device in mechanical thrombectomy led to the first U.S. Food and Drug Administration (FDA) approval of a thrombus extraction device for acute ischemic stroke in 2004. After early trial results demonstrated the technical feasibility of endovascular

Department of Neurosurgery, Icahn School of Medicine at Mount Sinai Hospital, 1 Gustave Levy Place, Annenberg Building 8th Floor, New York, NY 10029, USA
* Corresponding author.
E-mail address: kurt.yaeger@mountsinai.org
Twitter: @Dr_Yaeger (K.Y.)

Neurosurg Clin N Am 33 (2022) 233–239
https://doi.org/10.1016/j.nec.2021.11.007

thrombectomy,[3] the first randomized trials published in 2013 failed to observe a benefit in its primary outcome. Yet despite these findings, clinical, real-world success drove interventionalists to again innovate on existing stent-retriever devices (initially developed as aneurysm coil buttresses) and push for new trials with updated technology.[4] This ultimately resulted in the publication of several studies in 2015 demonstrating the clear efficacy of endovascular thrombectomy for patients with LVO, supported by level IA evidence in the most recent American Stroke Association (ASA) acute ischemic stroke guidelines.[5] From there, technical innovation in stent-retrievers,[6] aspiration catheters,[7] guidewires, and guide catheters[8] has continued to expand the armamentarium, allowing interventionalists to treat more patients quickly, safely, and effectively.

While innovation in device technology facilitated the development of endovascular thrombectomy for acute ischemic stroke, it also opened the field to consider additional new diseases that may be improved through endovascular means. For instance, there has been a philosophic shift among neurosurgeons and interventionalists that has ushered in an era of endovascular treatment of chronic subdural hematoma (cSDH). Traditionally, cSDH has been a difficult to manage condition, often affecting elderly and comorbid patients for whom surgical evacuation carries risks. Furthermore, there is up to 25% risk of cSDH recurrence after evacuation, further complicating existing surgical strategies.[9] However, a growing body of evidence has supported the use of middle meningeal artery (MMA) embolization for both cSDH treatment and recurrence prevention. Initial angiographic observations of increased and abnormal MMA vascularity of membranous cSDH spawned initial innovation for the endovascular treatment, which paved the way for early case reports and clinical trials.[10] The push by interventionalists to treat cSDH with the less invasive endovascular approach has demonstrated clinical promise: recent meta-analytical data suggests lower recurrence rates compared with surgical evacuation.[11] This has laid the foundation for ongoing randomized clinical trials, as this treatment strategy gains clinical acceptance.[12] Like endovascular thrombectomy for LVO, technical innovation has driven the adoption of a novel treatment paradigm for a complicated pathology, which has been supported by rigorous clinical research.

The innovation driving endovascular thrombectomy and MMA embolization are examples of how neurointerventionalists are driving the field forward. The trend of identifying a troubling pathology, innovating novel endovascular devices, and performing clinical research to support the innovation continues to be a hallmark of this field. The unknowns of endovascular neurosurgery are limited by the available technology, but there have been recent notable technical developments that herald the future of minimally invasive neurosurgical care: stent-based electrodes for functional motor deficits, endovascular treatment strategy for hydrocephalus, and innovations in the treatment of wide-neck intracranial aneurysms (WNAs).

ENDOVASCULAR STENT-ELECTRODE (STENTRODE)

Brain–computer interfaces (BCIs) have evolved from science fiction to reality over the past several decades. This broad category of technologies connects human neural activity to an external output device, such as a computer monitor, robotic arm, or artificial limb.[13] The clinical goal of these technologies is to bypass lesions in the corticospinal tracts such as stroke, spinal cord injury, and severe neurodegenerative diseases such as amyotrophic lateral sclerosis (ALS). Traditionally, these technologies consist of a sensory limb that detects neural impulses, a decoder that detects and decodes neural information, and effector limb that carries out the desires output function. Neural sensor devices vary widely in structure, invasiveness, and both spatial and temporal discrimination. On one end, a noninvasive scalp electroencephalogram (EEG) can be used to detect a broad region of neural circuitry, whereas on the other end, implanted microelectrode arrays can be used to detect highly specific neural networks with high resolution.[13] In general, temporal resolution of a BCI sensor increases with invasiveness, with scalp EEG resolution 50 ms than 3 ms for intraparenchymal microelectrodes, given the proximity to the neural circuitry and lack of signal degrading features such as bone or dural artifacts. As these invasive modalities are the fastest for interpreting neural activity, they make the most effective sensory limb for a BCI circuit, and the most likely to be incorporated for clinical use. However, as these modalities often require surgical implantation, there are inherent risks such as bleeding, infection, and sensor malpositioning.[14,15] Furthermore, chronic parenchymal implants are associated with inflammation and gliosis around the electrode site, which limits efficacy over time.[16]

Within the last decade, much work has been done to improve the temporospatial discrimination of BCI sensors, enhancing biocompatibility while limiting the invasiveness of implantation. Intracranial intravenous electroencephalography (EEG) was first experimented in patients with intractable epilepsy, with the goal of developing a less invasive intracranial EEG modality.[17] Given that veins typically lie in sulcal folds and deep cortical regions, the intracranial venous system was thought to represent an ideal avenue for long-term monitoring of neural activity, with access to brain regions inaccessible by surface electrodes. Further, by implanting electrodes within the venous system, these difficult to access regions can be monitored safely, without risks inherent to open surgical implantation. A recent systematic review of endovascular BCI resulted in 22 papers published on the topic between 1973 and 2018, with than half (12) published since 2010.[18] Most of the early studies were published in the 1990s, recognized the potential of endovascular EEG, and were performed as proof-of-concept studies and feasibility trials. However, the concept of using intravascular EEG as the sensory limb of a BCI circuit is relatively novel.

In 2016, Oxley and colleagues published a preliminary report on the use of a novel transvenous stent-electrode (Stentrode) for the use of chronic monitoring of sensorimotor cortical neural activity.[19] This self-expanding electrode array is capable of being delivered via catheter angiography through the superior sagittal sinus to cortical veins proximate to the sensorimotor cortex. The first Stentrode device was built using a commercially available intracranial nitinol stent-retriever (Solitaire, Medtronic, Ireland) as a scaffold for platinum disc electrodes, with electrode leads passing proximally along the stent wire. The electrodes were arranged coaxially around the stent tines to oppose the vessel wall after endovascular deployment. The Stentrodes were percutaneously inserted via common jugular vein access, and following implantation, the proximal leads were tunneled to an external receiver near the sternocleidomastoid muscle, for attachment to decoding hardware.

In their first animal trials, Oxley and coauthors assessed the efficacy of the Stentrode in sheep, and assessed vessel patency, impedance, and neural signal recording over a period of 3 months. A further cohort of sheep was used to validate the Stentrode signal against intracranial electrocorticography (ECoG) electrode arrays. Overall, the study confirmed the overall feasibility of endovascularly implanted transvenous electrodes, with several notable observations. First, the implant was appropriately incorporated into the vessel wall via endothelialization, and that changes to impedance values suggested that this process occurred within 6 days after implantation. Second, using somatosensory evoked potentials (SSEPs), the investigators determined that the Stentrode accurately measured cerebral activity from direct median nerve stimulation, and that the recording sensitivity increased over the first several days postimplantation. Next, localization of the motor cortex was able to be determined by phase reversal between electrodes on the stent. Lastly, the group observed chronic patency of the stent, assessing 20 sheep after 120 with the stent implanted. Despite the animals being on aspirin antiplatelet therapy, some of the cortical veins thrombosed in 3 of 8 total subjects after 3 months, albeit without any focal neurologic consequences. Altogether, these observations highlighted the feasibility and safety for implantation of an intracranial stent for the long-term monitoring of neural activity, setting the stage for first in human trials.

In October 2020, Oxley and colleagues published the results of their first-in-human trial, consisting of 2 subjects with ALS in whom the Stentrode BCI system was implanted for use controlling a mouse click on the computer screen.[20] Initiated in Australia, the trial was designed as a prospective, single-arm, open-label study assessing the safety and feasibility of the Stentrode BCI system. The human system is based on a custom self-expanding stent with 16 electrodes circumferentially ordered around the nitinol stent scaffolding (**Fig. 1**). The electrodes are connected to an intravascular lead, which is subsequently tunneled out the internal jugular vein and connected to a telemetry unit implanted above the pectoral muscle. An external telemetry unit wirelessly receives signal from the implanted device and relays it to a decoder, which processes the information to a commercially available tablet device. After system implantation, subjects underwent a training period, followed by a supervised performance testing, then unsupervised home use, which began at days 86 and 71 for the 2 subjects, respectively. Motor mapping was performed during initial training sessions and neural activity was decoded via use of a machine learning algorithm. Subjects were given a battery of motor activities prompted by on-screen cues. Computer mouse cursor was controlled using an eye movement tracker and click functionality was generated by the subjects' neural activity.

Both subjects underwent uneventful procedures, without significant complications, and follow-up imaging showed patency of the superior sagittal sinus at last follow-up for both patients. Click accuracy was determined to be 95% and 94% for the subjects following training. Furthermore, on independent performance, both subjects were able to carry out activities of daily living

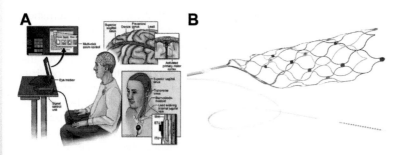

Fig. 1. Schematic of the Stentrode endovascular BCI system (Synchron, Melbourne, Australia). (*A*) The stent-based electrode array is implanted in the superior sagittal sinus near the region of the motor cortex. The lead is tunneled out of the internal jugular vein in the neck and connected to an internal telemetry unit (ITU), which is implanted in the chest. The signal is relayed wirelessly to an external telemetry unit (ETU), which is decoded and relayed to the computer as a signal output. (*B*) A depiction of the Stentrode device, with electrodes mounted radially around the self-expanding nitinol stent, intending to oppose the venous sinus, and become incorporated into the vessel wall. (Published with permission from the authors and Synchron.)

(ADLs) such as texting, emailing, and online shopping.

These studies represent a significant leap in endovascular neurosurgery, that of functional brain modulation facilitated by an endovascularly-delivered device. Given that most current BCI technologies require intracranial implantation to achieve the spatial and temporal fidelity required for functional use, the venous stent-electrode may represent a more feasible, long-term solution for recording neural activity, be it for responsive stimulation for epilepsy, BCI afferent signal for neurodegeneration, or other to-be-determined pathologic states. The future of endovascular BCI is clear: as latency improves, more complex mechanical output can be achieved, such as with mechanical arms or legs, expanding the indications to spinal cord injury or poststroke weakness.

ENDOVASCULAR TREATMENT OF HYDROCEPHALUS (eShunt)

Hydrocephalus has long been a challenging aspect of the neurosurgeon's practice. For years, surgeons have relied on surgical methods for relieving cerebrospinal fluid (CSF) outflow aberrations caused by either mechanical obstruction (noncommunicating hydrocephalus) or CSF reabsorption issues (communicating hydrocephalus). Initial surgical approaches described in the 1880s involved craniotomy and open ventricular drainage, which evolved to burr hole ventriculostomy placement, conceptualized in the 1940s.[21] Ventricular shunting was further developed to treat chronic hydrocephalus, yet involved implantation of foreign objects, leading to risks of infection, and mechanical failure. Using endoscopy to perform a third ventriculostomy (ETV) as an alternative treatment of obstructive hydrocephalus evolved as a less invasive method of CSF diversion, yet it still requires burr hole access and a transcortical approach to the ventricular system.

Despite advances in modern technology, the principles and devices of CSF diversion have remained overall consistent. The biggest innovations have come in the form of shunt catheter impregnation with antimicrobial substances and the innovation of programmable shunt valves. The introduction of antibiotic ventricular catheters has decreased the overall risk of shunt infection, rates of which vary but exceeds 12% in some studies.[22,23] Programmable valves allow the rate of CSF flow to depend on patient-specific factors, and titration based on symptoms or radiographic findings. But despite these technological improvements, shunts are still prone to mechanical failure that often requires revision and replacement.[24] This, in turn, leads to patient morbidity as well as increased costs of care. Certainly, hydrocephalus is pathology ripe for innovation and disruption.

Recently, Heilman and colleagues published a report documenting the anatomic relationships between the inferior petrosal sinus (IPS) and the cerebellopontine angle (CPA) cistern, identifying this relationship as a possible site for endovascular creation of a CSF-venous fistula for CSF diversion.[25] This novel concept leverages the positive pressure gradient between CSF and the cerebral venous system, and in essence, creates an artificial arachnoid granulation for CSF reuptake. The investigators have developed an endovascular system for creating this CSF-venous fistula, capable of being deployed into the CPA cistern from the IPS via a transvenous approach. They identified an ideal location for deployment, in the CPA cistern at the level of the jugular tubercle (**Fig. 2**). The eShunt device is implanted by puncturing the IPS at this location and deploying a valve within the cistern that drains CSF into the IPS

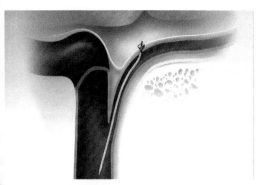

Fig. 2. The eShunt system (Cerevasc, Massachusetts, USA) is intended to bridge the fluid pressure gradient between cerebrospinal fluid (CSF) in the cerebello-pontine angle cistern and the venous blood in the inferior petrosal sinus as a treatment of hydrocephlaus. It is deployed by a microcatheter into the CPA cistern via a transvenous route. (Published with permission from Cerevasc.)

across the dura.[26] This solution may obviate the need for transcranial approaches for CSF diversion, limiting the open surgical complications, as well as complications associated with shunt catheters and valves. While more data are certainly warranted, the eShunt system represents a novel trajectory into the endovascular treatment of hydrocephalus.

ENDOVASCULAR TREATMENT OF WIDE-NECK INTRACRANIAL ANEURYSMS

WNAs represent a broad morphologic class of aneurysms that have traditionally been difficult to treat with both microsurgical and endovascular techniques. A recent systematic review observed that, while the definition of wide-neck is variable, most studies define the morphology as either neck greater than 4 mm or dome-to-neck ratio of less than 2, and recommended using these definitions for more consistent assessment across the literature.[27] Current endovascular treatment options include flow diversion or buttressed coil embolization with stent, balloon, or neck-support device. More recently, intra-saccular devices have emerged as promising treatment options for WNAs. However, there is certainly no standard treatment approach for these aneurysms, and there are varying occlusion rates using these devices. In one multi-institutional, core-lab adjudicated study of endovascularly treated WNAs, the occlusion rate (RR1) at follow-up was 30.6%, with a short-term retreatment rate of 8.7%.[28] The authors concluded that more innovation in

endovascular devices will be key in expanding the window for successful treatment in patients with WNAs. Over the past few years, innovation in this space has expanded, specifically with intra-saccular devices and deployable coil buttresses, laying the groundwork for improved safety and efficacy for the endovascular treatment of WNAs.

The first long-term results of the first deployable intrasaccular device were released in 2019 by the WEB-IT study investigators.[29] This group assessed the efficacy and safety of the Woven EndoBridge (WEB, Microvention, USA) device for patients with WNAs. The WEB is a self-expanding, 3-dimensional basket, constructed using braided nitinol and platinum wires, and developed specifically for deployment in WNAs. In 148 patients, the researchers observed a 12-month complete occlusion (RR1) rate of 53.8% and acceptable occlusion rates (RR1/2) of 84.6%. Furthermore, only 1 primary safety event was noted up to 12-months follow-up: that of a spontaneous, ipsilateral intracerebral hematoma.

As the conclusion of the WEB-IT trial, 2 novel devices have emerged as alternative endovascular treatment modalities for WNAs. The first is the Contour device (Cerus Endovascular, USA), a nitinol mesh basket that is deployed within the neck of a WNA to perform as a flow diverter as well as flow disruptor to facilitate blood stasis within the aneurysm dome. In a single-center feasibility study, the Contour device was deployed in 11 patients with WNAs.[30] The authors observed a complete occlusion rate (RR1) of 55.6% and all patients had at least an acceptable aneurysmal occlusion (RR1/2). However, 2 patients experienced distal thromboembolic events following the procedure, but neither had long-term disability at follow-up. The second novel device is the Nautilus device (EndoStream Medical, Israel), a spiraled, self-expanding nitinol wire implant used for intrasaccular coil support. This implant was developed for patients with WNA and a contraindication for dual antiplatelet therapy. Recently, Sirakov and colleagues published the first case report using the Nautilus device in a patient with WNA.[31] The authors documented the feasibility of the device deployment and observed its unique "tornado shape" reconstructing the aneurysm neck temporarily while embolic coils were implanted in the aneurysm sac. Overall, the investigators of both devices acknowledge that more research is certainly needed, but the results are encouraging for using the Contour and Nautilus as alternative treatment strategies for WNA embolization, thus paving the way for the treatment of aneurysms not conventionally treated by endovascular techniques.

SUMMARY

It is clear that the field of endovascular neurosurgery has been, and is continuously, forward thinking with regard to innovating on behalf of patients with diseases previously considered difficult, if not impossible, to treat effectively. Our ability to treat different aneurysms, AVMs, and strokes have been amplified by advances in device technology, making these pathologies more accessible and safer to treat. Presently, we are bordering on paradigm-shifting endovascular technology that facilitates treatment of not simply cerebrovascular disease, but nonvascular disease states such as neurodegeneration and hydrocephalus. For endovascular BCI, as the technology improves, more complex motor output can be achieved, with the goal of using neural signals to control mechanical arms or legs. One can postulate other neurologic diseases that, as of yet, have no routine endovascular treatment options, such as intrinsic tumors, infectious processes, and intractable headaches, that may be grounds for innovation in the coming years. Innovation, collaboration, device development, industry partnership, and research support are essential factors for growth in endovascular neurosurgery and facilitate forward progress within this specialty on behalf of our patients.

CLINICS CARE POINTS

- The list of neuropathologies treated by endovascular means continues to expand.
- The specialty is driven to innovate by both clinicians and industry.
- The future of hydrocephalus management as well as functional neurosurgery has promise with endovascular techniques.
- The more distant future of what is possible with neuroendovascular management is ripe for further innovation.

CONFLICTS OF INTEREST

K. Yaeger: none. J. Mocco: Investor in BlinkTBI, Cerebrotech, Comet, Echovate, Endostream, Imperative Care, NTI Managers, Radical, Serenity, Synchron, Viz.ai; Consultant for CVAid, Perflow, Viz.ai.

REFERENCES

1. Tissue plasminogen activator for acute ischemic stroke. N Engl J Med 1995;333(24):1581–8.
2. Smith W, Furlan A. Brief history of endovascular acute ischemic stroke treatment. Stroke 2016; 47(2):e23–6.
3. Smith WS, Sung G, Starkman S, et al. Safety and Efficacy of Mechanical Embolectomy in Acute Ischemic Stroke. Stroke 2005;36(7):1432–8.
4. Boyle K, Joundi RA, Aviv RI. An historical and contemporary review of endovascular therapy for acute ischemic stroke. Neurovascular Imaging 2017;3(1):1–12.
5. Powers WJ, Rabinstein AA, Ackerson T, et al. 2018 guidelines for the early management of patients with acute ischemic stroke: a guideline for healthcare professionals from the American Heart Association/American Stroke Association. Stroke 2018; 49(3):e46–110.
6. Zaidat OO, Bozorgchami H, Ribó M, et al. Primary results of the multicenter ARISE II study (analysis of revascularization in ischemic stroke with embotrap). Stroke 2018;49(5):1107–15.
7. Turk A, Siddiqui A, Fifi J, et al. Aspiration thrombectomy versus stent retriever thrombectomy as first-line approach for large vessel occlusion (COMPASS): a multicentre, randomised, open label, blinded outcome, non-inferiority trial. Lancet 2019; 393(10175):998–1008.
8. Bageac DV, Gershon BS, Vargas J, et al. Comparative study of intracranial access in thrombectomy using next generation 0.088 inch guide catheter technology. J Neurointerv Surg 2021;1–7. https://doi.org/10.1136/NEURINTSURG-2021-017341.
9. Sahyouni R, Goshtasbi K, Mahmoodi A, et al. Chronic subdural hematoma: a historical and clinical perspective. World Neurosurg 2017;108:948–53.
10. Mandai S, Sakurai M, Matsumoto Y. Middle meningeal artery embolization for refractory chronic subdural hematoma. Case report. J Neurosurg 2000; 93(4):686–8.
11. Srivatsan A, Mohanty A, Nascimento F, et al. Middle Meningeal Artery Embolization for Chronic Subdural Hematoma: Meta-Analysis and Systematic Review. World Neurosurg 2019;122:613–9.
12. Moshayedi P, Liebeskind DS. Middle Meningeal Artery Embolization in Chronic Subdural Hematoma: Implications of Pathophysiology in Trial Design. Front Neurol 2020;11. https://doi.org/10.3389/FNEUR.2020.00923.
13. Martini ML, Oermann EK, Opie NL, et al. Sensor Modalities for Brain-Computer Interface Technology: A Comprehensive Literature Review. Clin Neurosurg 2020;86(2). https://doi.org/10.1093/neuros/nyz286.
14. Bjornsson C, Oh S, Al-Kofahi Y, et al. Effects of insertion conditions on tissue strain and vascular damage during neuroprosthetic device insertion. J Neural Eng 2006;3(3):196–207.
15. Leuthardt E, Moran D, Mullen T. Defining Surgical Terminology and Risk for Brain Computer Interface

Technologies. Front Neurosci 2021;15. https://doi.org/10.3389/FNINS.2021.599549.

16. Karumbaiah L, Saxena T, Carlson D, et al. Relationship between intracortical electrode design and chronic recording function. Biomaterials 2013; 34(33):8061–74.

17. Boniface SJ, Antoun N. Endovascular electroencephalography: the technique and its application during carotid amytal assessment. J Neurol Neurosurg Psychiatry 1997;62(2):193–5.

18. Soldozy S, Young S, Kumar JS, et al. A systematic review of endovascular stent-electrode arrays, a minimally invasive approach to brain-machine interfaces. Neurosurg Focus 2020;49(1):E3.

19. Oxley TJ, Opie NL, John SE, et al. Minimally invasive endovascular stent-electrode array for high-fidelity, chronic recordings of cortical neural activity. Nat Biotechnol 2016;34(3):320–7.

20. Oxley T, Yoo P, Rind G, et al. Motor neuroprosthesis implanted with neurointerventional surgery improves capacity for activities of daily living tasks in severe paralysis: first in-human experience. J Neurointerv Surg 2021;13(2):102–8.

21. Demerdash A, Rocque BG, Johnston J, et al. Endoscopic third ventriculostomy: A historical review. Br J Neurosurg 2016;31(1):28–32.

22. Stevens N, Greene C, O'Gara J, et al. Ventriculoperitoneal shunt-related infections caused by Staphylococcus epidermidis: pathogenesis and implications for treatment. Br J Neurosurg 2012;26(6):792–7.

23. Konstantelias A, Vardakas K, Polyzos K, et al. Antimicrobial-impregnated and -coated shunt catheters for prevention of infections in patients with hydrocephalus: a systematic review and meta-analysis. J Neurosurg 2015;122(5):1096–112.

24. Jorgensen J, Williams C, Sarang-Sieminski A. Hydrocephalus and Ventriculoperitoneal Shunts: Modes of Failure and Opportunities for Improvement. Crit Rev Biomed Eng 2016;44(1–2):91–7.

25. Heilman CB, Basil GW, Beneduce BM, et al. Anatomical characterization of the inferior petrosal sinus and adjacent cerebellopontine angle cistern for development of an endovascular transdural cerebrospinal fluid shunt. J Neurointerv Surg 2019;11(6):598–602.

26. Minimally invasive treatment of hydrocephalus | CereVasc. Available at: https://cerevasc.com/treatment-of-hydrocephalus/. Accessed October 7, 2021.

27. Hendricks BK, Yoon JS, Yaeger K, et al. Wide-neck aneurysms: systematic review of the neurosurgical literature with a focus on definition and clinical implications. J Neurosurg 2019;133(1):159–65.

28. De Leacy R, Fargen K, Mascitelli J, et al. Wide-neck bifurcation aneurysms of the middle cerebral artery and basilar apex treated by endovascular techniques: a multicentre, core lab adjudicated study evaluating safety and durability of occlusion (BRANCH). J Neurointerv Surg 2019;11(1):31–6.

29. Arthur AS, Molyneux A, Coon AL, et al. The safety and effectiveness of the woven endobridge (web) system for the treatment of wide-necked bifurcation aneurysms: Final 12-month results of the pivotal web intrasaccular therapy (web-it) study. J Neurointerv Surg 2019;11(9):924–30.

30. Akhunbay-Fudge CY, Deniz K, Tyagi AK, et al. Endovascular treatment of wide-necked intracranial aneurysms using the novel Contour Neurovascular System: A single-center safety and feasibility study. J Neurointerv Surg 2020;12(10):987–92.

31. Sirakov A, Matanov S, Bhogal P, et al. Nautilus-assisted coil embolization for a complex AcomA wide-necked aneurysm in the setting of acute subarachnoid hemorrhage. J Neurointerv Surg 2021. https://doi.org/10.1136/NEURINTSURG-2021-017670. neurintsurg-2021-017670.

Moving?

Make sure your subscription moves with you!

To notify us of your new address, find your **Clinics Account Number** (located on your mailing label above your name), and contact customer service at:

Email: journalscustomerservice-usa@elsevier.com

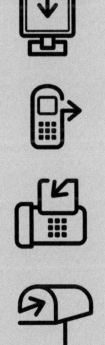

800-654-2452 (subscribers in the U.S. & Canada)
314-447-8871 (subscribers outside of the U.S. & Canada)

Fax number: 314-447-8029

Elsevier Health Sciences Division
Subscription Customer Service
3251 Riverport Lane
Maryland Heights, MO 63043

*To ensure uninterrupted delivery of your subscription, please notify us at least 4 weeks in advance of move.

Printed and bound by CPI Group (UK) Ltd, Croydon, CR0 4YY

08/05/2025

01864713-0008